ADVANCES IN

Vascular Surgery

VOLUME 1

ADVANCES IN

Vascular Surgery

VOLUME 1

Editor-in Chief
Anthony D. Whittemore, M.D.
Associate Professor Surgery, Harvard University Medical School; Chief,
Division of Vascular Surgery, Brigham and Women's Hospital, Boston,
Massachusetts

Associate Editors
Dennis F. Bandyk, M.D.
Professor of Surgery, University of South Florida College of Medicine; Director,
Vascular Surgery Division, Chief of Vascular Surgery, Tampa General Hospital,
Tampa, Florida

Jack L. Cronenwett, M.D.
Professor of Surgery, Dartmouth College, Mary Hitchcock Medical Center,
Hanover, New Hampshire

Norman R. Hertzer, M.D.
Chairman, Department of Vascular Surgery, Cleveland Clinic Foundation,
Cleveland, Ohio

Rodney A. White, M.D.
Professor of Surgery, University of California at Los Angeles School of
Medicine; Chief of Vascular Surgery, Harbor–University of California at Los
Angeles Medical Center, Los Angeles, California

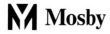 Mosby

St. Louis Baltimore Boston Chicago London Madrid Philadelphia Sydney Toronto

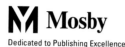

Mosby

Dedicated to Publishing Excellence

Sponsoring Editor: Linda M. Steiner
Project Manager: Denise Dungey
Project Supervisor: Maria Nevinger
Production Editor: Laura Pelehach
Staff Support Administrator: Barbara M. Kelly

Editorial Office:
Mosby–Year Book, Inc.
200 North LaSalle St.
Chicago, IL 60601

International Standard Serial Number: 1069-7292
International Standard Book Number: 0-8151-9405-6

Contributors

Samuel C. Aldridge, M.D.
Instructor of Surgery, Temple University School of Medicine; Clinical Vascular Surgery Fellow, Temple University Hospital, Philadelphia, Pennsylvania

Michael Belkin, M.D.
Assistant Professor of Surgery, Tufts University School of Medicine; New England Medical Center Hospital, Boston, Massachusetts

Anthony J. Comerota, M.D.
Professor of Surgery, Temple University School of Medicine; Chief of Vascular Surgery, Temple University Hospital, Philadelphia, Pennsylvania

Douglas M. Cavaye, M.D., B.S., F.R.A.C.S.
Instructor in Surgery, University of California at Los Angeles School of Medicine; Vascular Surgeon, Harbor–University of California at Los Angeles Medical Center, Los Angeles, California

Richard H. Dean, M.D.
Professor and Director, Division of Surgical Sciences, Bowman Gray School of Medicine, Wake Forest University, Winston-Salem, North Carolina

Magruder C. Donaldson, M.D.
Assistant Professor of Surgery, Harvard Medical School; Brigham and Women's Hospital, Boston, Massachusetts

Carlos Encarnacion, M.D.
Assistant Professor, Department of Radiology, The University of Texas Health Sciences Center, San Antonio, Texas

Calvin B. Ernst, M.D.
Clinical Professor of Surgery, University of Michigan Medical School, Ann Arbor; Head, Division of Vascular Surgery, Henry Ford Hospital, Detroit, Michigan

Robert W. Hobson II, M.D.
Professor of Surgery; Chief, Section of Vascular Surgery, University of Medicine and Dentistry of New Jersey, New Jersey Medical School, Newark, New Jersey

Larry H. Hollier, M.D.
Chairman, Department of Surgery, Ochsner Clinic and Alton Ochsner Medical Foundation; Clinical Professor of Surgery, Louisiana State University School of Medicine and Tulane University Medical Center, New Orleans, Louisiana

Thomas C. Naslund, M.D.
Assistant Professor of Surgery, Division of Vascular Surgery, Vanderbilt University Medical Center, Nashville, Tennessee

Kevin D. Nolan, M.D., M.P.H.
Instructor of Surgery, Division of Vascular Surgery, Northwestern University Medical School, Chicago, Illinois

Julio C. Palmaz, M.D.
Professor, Department of Radiology; Chief, Cardiovascular and Special Interventions, The University of Texas Health Science Center, San Antonio, Texas

Juan C. Parodi, M.D.
Assistant Professor of Surgery, Universidad del Salvador; Chairman, Department of Vascular Surgery, Instituto Cardiovascular de Buenos Aires, Buenos Aires, Argentina

William H. Pearce, M.D.
Associate Professor of Surgery, Division of Vascular Surgery, Northwestern University Medical Center, Chicago, Illinois

Frank J. Rivera, M.D.
Assistant Professor, Department of Radiology, The University of Texas Health Sciences Center, San Antonio, Texas

Alexander D. Shepard, M.D.
Clinical Assistant Professor of Surgery, University of Michigan Medical School, Ann Arbor; Senior Staff Surgeon, Division of Vascular Surgery, Henry Ford Hospital, Detroit, Michigan

D. Eugene Strandness, Jr., M.D.
Professor and Chief, Division of Vascular Surgery, University of Washington School of Medicine; Attending Vascular Surgeon, University of Washington Medical Center, Seattle, Washington

Jesse E. Thompson, M.D.
Clinical Professor of Surgery, University of Texas Southwestern Medical School; Former Chief of Surgery and Vascular Surgery, Baylor University Medical Center, Dallas, Texas

Rodney A. White, M.D.
Professor of Surgery, University of California at Los Angeles School of Medicine; Chief of Vascular Surgery, Harbor–University of California at Los Angeles Medical Center, Los Angeles, California

James S.T. Yao, M.D., Ph.D.
Magerstadt Professor of Surgery, Department of Surgery, Division of Vascular Surgery, Northwestern University Medical School, Chicago, Illinois

R. Eugene Zierler, M.D.
Associate Professor of Surgery, University of Washington School of Medicine, Seattle, Washington

Preface

This inaugural volume of *Advances in Vascular Surgery* represents the most recent addition to the publisher's well-received specialty series. The editorial board seeks to provide vascular surgeons, nurses, and technicians with a annual scholarly review of evolving concepts that have recently modified or that show potential for altering current clinical approaches to specific vascular entities. The board consists of practicing vascular surgeons with acknowledged expertise in various aspects of clinical vascular surgery as well as in specific areas of investigative endeavor.

While it is our intent to present timely coverage of a variety of subjects, it is also useful to emphasize one particular area in more detail each year. With the publication of the North American Carotid Endarterectomy Trial, its European counterpart, and the multicenter VA Clinical Trial, it seems only appropriate to focus on intervention for extracranial vascular disease in this first edition. Each year we will select an individual whose outstanding contributions have shaped the evolution of our current approach to this focused area. Dr. Jesse Thompson has remained an extraordinarily articulate advocate of carotid endarterectomy since its inception, and we are indebted to him for providing an enlightening introductory chapter. Drs. Strandness and Hobson have been intimately involved with the ongoing clinical trials for symptomatic and asymptomatic carotid disease and have submitted detailed reviews of the recent data that guide our current strategies. Dr. Zierler has contributed a thorough review of his perspectives on the evaluation of carotid disease, a rapidly evolving field in which he has been instrumental.

The remaining chapters address current topics in aortic reconstruction, endovascular techniques, thrombolytic therapy, and important changes with respect to indications for intervention in renovascular disease and methods for reconstruction.

The final chapter in each volume will be devoted to some aspect of basic scientific investigation or pathophysiology whose impact on clinical practice appears near at hand. In this volume Dr. Donaldson has elaborated on the hypercoagulable states and describes an approach toward dealing with the potential impact of the more commonly encountered hypercoagulopathies.

It is the sincere hope of the publishers and editorial board that our goals will be consistently met and in so doing provide the clinical vascular surgeon with a scholarly approach toward solving clinical problems encountered in the evolving practice of our specialty.

Anthony D. Whittemore, M.D.

Contents

PART I

Carotid Artery Disease

Historical Perspective of Carotid Artery Disease

JESSE E. THOMPSON, M.D.

C hanging concepts of the etiology, diagnosis, and treatment of ischemic stroke syndromes in the past 40 years have been responsible for widespread renewal of interest in this disease. Increasing awareness of the extracranial location and segmental nature of atherosclerotic occlusive disease in a large proportion of patients with cerebrovascular insufficiency was followed by the development and employment of appropriate vascular surgical techniques for removing or bypassing offending plaques, thus increasing cerebral blood flow or eliminating sources of cerebral emboli. Since extracranial carotid lesions are those encountered most frequently, surgery of the carotid artery has become a subject of heightened interest and importance. In fact, carotid endarterectomy now is the most frequently performed peripheral vascular operation in the United States. It is the purpose of this chapter to review the historical background of carotid artery surgery as it relates to the management of cerebrovascular insufficiency.[1, 2]

The word "carotid" is derived from the Greek term *karotide* or *karos*, meaning to stupefy or plunge into deep sleep. According to Rufus of Ephesus (circa A.D. 100), the term was applied to the arteries of the neck because compression of these vessels produced stupor or sleep.[1] Figure 1 is a photo of the 31st metope from the south side of the Parthenon in Athens, now safely ensconced in the British Museum among the Elgin Marbles, which demonstrates that the ancient Greeks were aware of the significance of the carotid artery, with a centaur applying left carotid compression to the neck of a Lapith warrior. According to Dandy, Hippocrates (460 to 370 B.C.) and Galen (A.D. 131 to 201) were aware that hemiplegia resulted from a lesion in the opposite side of the brain.[3]

Ambroise Paré in the 16th century was familiar with the carotid phenomenon and stated, "The two branches they call carotides or soporales, the sleepy arteries, because they being obstructed or any way stopt we presently fall asleep."[4]

Johann Jakob Wepfer, a Swiss physician, in 1658 was the first to describe carotid thrombosis, extracranially and intracranially, in a patient with a completely occluded and calcified right internal carotid artery. In his *Apoplexia*, he traced the carotid and vertebral arteries from their origins to the arterial circle at the base of the brain and noted that apoplexy could result from cerebral hemorrhage.[5, 6]

According to Cutter,[7] Jean Luis Petit in the 18th century discovered

Advances in Vascular Surgery, vol. 1.
©1993, Mosby–Year Book, Inc.

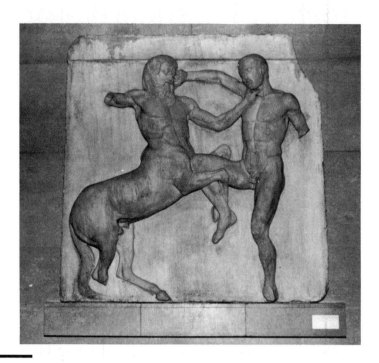

FIGURE 1.

The 31st metope from the Parthenon, showing a centaur applying carotid compression to the neck of a Lapith warrior. (Photograph by the author in the British Museum.)

that the brain may survive deprived of the contribution of one carotid artery. His patient had an aneurysm of the bifurcation of the right common carotid artery that underwent spontaneous cure. Seven years later, autopsy showed the lumen of the vessel to be occluded completely by organized thrombus.[8]

The first operations on the carotid artery were, quite naturally, ligation procedures for trauma or hemorrhage. Hebenstreit of Germany, in his translation of Benjamin Bell's *Surgery* in 1793, mentions a case in which the carotid artery was injured during operative removal of a scirrhous tumor. The surgeon ligated the vessel to arrest hemorrhage and the patient lived for many years. This is thought to be the first case on record of ligature of the carotid, although the exact date is not given.[7, 9, 10]

John Abernethy of London, a pupil of John Hunter, in 1804 reported a case of carotid ligation performed some years previously, probably in 1798, although the exact date cannot be ascertained. The patient, a man, was gored in the neck by the horn of a cow and hemorrhage was profuse. Compression controlled the bleeding temporarily, only to have it recur when pressure was released. Abernethy was compelled to ligate the common carotid artery. He states, "in attempting to secure the carotid artery I passed behind it . . . a blunt hook with an eye in the point, and having previously introduced a ligature into it I drew back the instrument and thus enclosed the artery." Hemorrhage was controlled and the patient appeared well. However, the man died 30 hours later of cerebral causes and Abernethy abandoned the procedure.[7, 10−12]

With the beginning of the 19th century, the history of carotid surgery becomes more accurate as dates of operations are given with exactness. The first successful ligation of a carotid artery was performed by David Fleming on October 17, 1803. David Fleming was a young naval surgeon aboard His Majesty's ship *Tonnant*, the greatest two-decker in the British navy, carrying 80 guns and cruising off the Spanish coast during the Napoleonic era. Mark Jackson, a servant, attempted to commit suicide by cutting his throat on October 9, 1803. The knife had grazed the outer and muscular coats of the carotid artery, but left the artery intact. Eight days later, on October 17, the carotid ruptured. Fleming cut down on the artery proximal to the rupture and ligated it. He had not done this before, nor had he heard of Abernethy's case. The patient survived and made an uninterrupted recovery. The case was reported in 1817 by Dr. Richard Warren Coley, an assistant surgeon on HMS *Tonnant*. This was the first *authentic* successful case of ligation of the carotid artery on record.[13, 14]

The first case of ligature of the carotid artery in the United States was that of Mason F. Cogswell of Hartford, Connecticut, performed November 4, 1803, the report being published in October of 1824. The patient, a 38-year-old woman, had an extensive tumor of the left side of her neck that completely enveloped the carotid artery. During the course of its removal, the carotid artery had to be ligated and divided. The patient did well at first, but on the 20th day, died as a result of hemorrhage from the wound. Cogswell stated, "the circumstances attending this case were such as entirely to establish the practicability and safety of dividing the carotid artery on the living subject."[7, 10, 15]

The first *successful* ligation of the carotid artery in the United States was done by Dr. Amos Twitchell of Keene, New Hampshire, on October 18, 1807. John Taggart, a cavalry soldier, age 20 years, in a mock fight at a regimental review, was wounded accidentally in the neck by a pistol shot on October 8, 1807. The wound was treated by simple dressings, although Dr. Twitchell commented, "there was a good deal of arterial excitement." Taggart improved rapidly, however, until the tenth day, when the internal carotid artery ruptured and "the blood jetted forcibly in a large stream to the distance of three or four feet." Twitchell stopped the hemorrhage by compression, then made an incision lower in the neck and ligated the common carotid artery with the patient's mother acting as his assistant. To his surprise, bleeding continued from the distal vessel. He then packed the wound tightly with dry sponges and the bleeding stopped. Fourteen days later, after all the packing was removed, the wound granulated in, and the patient made an uneventful recovery. This case was done 8 months prior to Astley Cooper's successful operation to be described below. At the time, Twitchell was ignorant of any other previous ligations of the carotid artery. The case was not reported until 1842, in the short-lived *New England Quarterly Journal of Medicine and Surgery*.* Amos Twitchell, who died in 1850, became the leading surgeon in his area of New England and performed all the major surgical operations of his day.[7, 16]

---

*This same volume contains the famous essay by Oliver Wendell Holmes on "The Contagiousness of Puerperal Fever."

Sir Astley Cooper in London was the first to attempt ligation of a carotid for cervical aneurysm on November 1, 1805. This patient died of sepsis on the 21st day with a left hemiparesis. Cooper repeated the operation on June 22, 1808, at Guy's Hospital. The patient was 55 years of age and had a pulsating tumor the size of an egg at the angle of the jaw. Two ligatures were applied to the artery, which was divided. The patient made a perfect recovery with no untoward symptoms and lived until 1821. This was the first successful case of ligature of the carotid artery for aneurysm.[17, 18]

The first successful ligation of the carotid for aneurysm in the United States was performed by Dr. Wright Post of New York City on January 9, 1813. After a stormy postoperative course, the patient finally survived.[10]

Benjamin Travers, on May 23, 1809, first successfully ligated the left carotid for carotid-cavernous fistula, with disappearance of signs and symptoms. In 1885, Victor Horsley first successfully ligated the carotid in the neck for an intracranial aneurysm. The patient was well 5 years later. By 1868, Pilz had been able to collect 600 recorded cases of carotid ligation for cervical aneurysm or hemorrhage, with a mortality rate of 43%.[12]

The American surgeon John Wyeth in 1878 published an extensive report detailing 898 collected cases of common carotid ligation. He found the mortality rate to be 41%, in contrast to that after ligature of the external carotid, which was only 4.5%.[19]

Until fairly recently, the prevailing notion held by most physicians was that strokes were caused by intracranial vascular disease. William Osler, in his textbook entitled *The Principles and Practice of Medicine* in the seventh edition of 1909 (the last edition that he himself wrote), attributed apoplectic stroke largely to cerebral hemorrhage. No mention is made of extracranial occlusive disease and, in the section dealing with cerebral softening, in which embolism and thrombosis are mentioned, emphasis is upon blockage of intracranial vessels.[20] This is somewhat curious in view of the fact that several authors already had described occlusive lesions in the extracranial segments of the main arteries supplying the brain and had noted their association with symptoms of cerebral ischemia.

William Heberden (1710 to 1801), a prominent London practitioner, had observed and described symptoms of transient cerebral insufficiency recurring in hours, days, or even months prior to the final episode of hemiplegia.[6, 21]

Gull, in 1855, had written of a case of occlusion of the innominate and left carotid.[22]

W. S. Savory, in 1856, published a landmark article on cerebral ischemia. In it, he described the case of a 22-year-old woman who had no pulsation in any of the vessels of the head, neck, or upper extremities. She had symptoms involving the left eye and right side of her body, both motor and sensory, as well as dizziness and convulsions. At postmortem examination, she had obliteration of the left carotid and both subclavian arteries. Savory commented on the relationship between the vascular occlusions and the clinical phenomena observed.[23]

In 1856, Virchow described carotid thrombosis associated with ipsilateral blindness, but found the lumens of the ophthalmic and central retinal arteries to be patent.[5]

Broadbent, in 1875, reported the case of a 50-year-old patient with absent pulses in both radial arteries. At autopsy, the origins of the innominate, left carotid, and subclavian arteries were constricted tightly, whereas the vessels distal to the narrowing appeared full and healthy.[24]

Penzoldt, in 1888, reported a case of thrombosis of the right common carotid artery. The patient developed a sudden permanent blindness in the right eye and later sustained a left hemiplegia. At autopsy, the right common carotid was thrombosed and the right cerebral hemisphere had a large area of softening.[25]

In 1905, Chiari described ulcerating plaques at the carotid bifurcation and, on the basis of detailed pathologic examinations, found that emboli could break away from carotid sinus–area plaques and cause strokes. He was among the first to propose that occlusive disease of the extracranial blood vessels could be responsible for neurologic symptoms.[6, 26]

Another landmark article was that of J. Ramsay Hunt of New York City in 1914, who called attention once again to the importance of extracranial occlusions in cerebrovascular disease. He recognized that both partial and complete occlusions of the innominate and carotid arteries could be responsible for cerebral syndromes of vascular origin and even used the term "cerebral intermittent claudication." He suggested that extracranial obstructions largely had been overlooked, and emphasized the importance of examining the cervical carotid system in patients with strokes. He also stressed "the occurrence of unilateral vascular changes, pallor or atrophy of the disk with contralateral hemiplegia in obstruction of the carotid artery."[27]

The next significant contribution was the report of Egas Móniz of Portugal, who, in 1927, first described the technique of cerebral arteriography and thus laid the groundwork of a practical method for the diagnosis of occlusive lesions.[28] The first report of carotid thrombosis demonstrated by arteriography was that of Sjöqvist in 1936.[29] The following year, 1937, Móniz, Lima, and de Lacerda reported four patients with occlusion of the cervical portion of the internal carotid artery in whom the diagnosis had been established by arteriography.[30] Egas Móniz won a Nobel Prize in 1949, not for cerebral arteriography, but for his work on prefrontal lobotomy.

Chao and associates in 1938 reported two cases similar to those of Móniz and colleagues.[31] By 1951, Johnson and Walker were able to collect from the literature 101 instances of carotid thrombosis, all diagnosed by this technique.[32]

In two important papers published in 1951 and 1954, C. Miller Fisher, working in Montreal but later in Boston, reemphasized the relationship between and frequency of disease of the carotid artery in the neck and cerebrovascular insufficiency. He defined the basic nature of the lesion as atherosclerosis, noted again partial and complete occlusions, and described severe syndromes associated with such occlusive disease. He observed that, with severe stenosis of the carotid bifurcation, the distal vessels could be entirely free of disease. He realized the importance of these observations, and stated:

it is even conceivable that some day vascular surgery will find a way to bypass the occluded portion of the artery during the period of ominous fleeting symptoms. Anastomosis of the external carotid artery or one of its branches with the internal carotid artery above the area of narrowing should be feasible.[33, 34]

Surgical methods of treating carotid artery occlusive disease prior to 1951 were (1) stellate ganglion block, (2) cervical sympathectomy, (3) removal of thrombi with reestablishment of blood flow, (4) ligation and excision of the carotid bifurcation, and (5) intracranial ligation of the carotid artery with silver clips. The reasons given for employing these methods were (1) the release of vasospasm in the vessels supplying the brain by interrupting periarterial sympathetics and (2) the prevention of forward embolism from clots in the cervical vessels.[35, 36]

In 1951, E. J. Wylie had introduced into the United States the procedure of thromboendarterectomy for the removal of atherosclerotic plaques from the aortoiliac segments, but it had not been employed on the carotid artery.[37]

Fisher's prophecy of surgical reconstruction of the carotid artery in the neck, as therapy for occlusive disease, soon was fulfilled. The first successful reconstruction of the carotid artery was performed by Carrea, Molins, and Murphy in Buenos Aires in 1951 after reading Fisher's article, and was reported in 1955.[38] A 41-year-old man had recurring symptoms of right hemiparesis, aphasia, and left amaurosis over a 6-month period before being referred to the neurologic and neurosurgical service of Dr. Raul Carrea by Dr. G. Murphy. Left percutaneous arteriography dem-

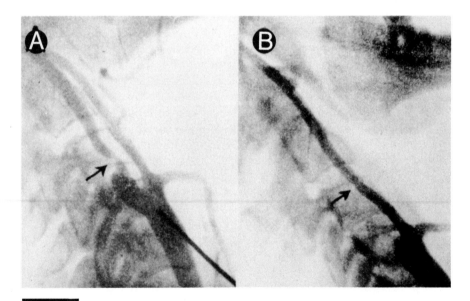

FIGURE 2.

A, preoperative arteriogram of the first carotid reconstruction case, done by Carrea, Molins, and Murphy in 1951. *Arrow* indicates the carotid lesion. B, postoperative arteriogram of the same case following anastomosis between the left external and internal carotid arteries after partial resection of the stenosed area. *Arrow* indicates site of anastomosis. (Courtesy of Dr. Patricio A. Welsh.)

onstrated an atherosclerotic plaque with severe stenosis in the internal carotid artery (Fig 2, A). On October 20, 1951, Dr. Molins, a vascular surgeon, and Dr. Carrea performed an end-to-end anastomosis between the left external carotid and the distal internal carotid arteries following partial resection of the stenosed area, together with cervical sympathectomy (see Fig 2, B). The patient made an uneventful recovery and was still alive and well 31 years following the operation except for loss of vision in the left eye.

On January 28, 1953, Strully, Hurwitt, and Blankenberg first attempted thromboendarterectomy of a totally occluded cervical internal carotid artery, but were unable to obtain retrograde flow. They suggested that endarterectomy should be feasible in such cases when the distal vasculature was patent.[39]

The first successful carotid endarterectomy was performed by Michael E. DeBakey on August 7, 1953. A 53-year-old school bus driver gave a history of recurring episodes of transient right hemiparesis and dysphasia over a 2-year period. On examination in August of 1953, he had a mild residual right hemiparesis and a weak pulsation in his left carotid artery. No preoperative arteriogram was done. At operation, a severely stenotic atherosclerotic plaque with superimposed fresh clot completely occluding the left internal carotid artery was found. Thromboendarterectomy was carried out, with good retrograde flow from both internal and external carotid arteries. An arteriogram performed postoperatively on the operating table showed the internal carotid to be patent in both its extracranial and intracranial portions. The patient made a good recovery and lived for 19 years without having further strokes. He died of complications of coronary artery disease August 17, 1972.[40]

The operation that gave the greatest impetus to the development of surgery for carotid occlusive disease was that of Eastcott, Pickering, and Rob performed on May 19, 1954, and reported in November of 1954.[41] In this case, a 66-year-old woman having suffered 33 transient episodes of right hemiparesis, aphasia, and left amaurosis over a 5-month period was found to have a severe stenosis of the left carotid bifurcation following a percutaneous left carotid arteriogram. Under general anesthesia with hypothermia to 28°C (82.4°F) for cerebral protection, the bifurcation was resected and blood flow restored by end-to-end anastomosis between the common carotid and distal internal carotid arteries. The carotid was occluded for 28 minutes. The patient was relieved of her symptoms completely and was alive and well at the age of 86 years. Figure 3 is an actual photograph taken during the performance of this historic operation at St. Mary's Hospital in London.

In February of 1956, Francis Murphey of Memphis, Tennessee performed successful carotid endarterectomies for both partial and total occlusions.[42]

On August 9, 1956, the late Champ Lyons accomplished a successful bypass from the right subclavian to the right carotid artery in the neck employing a nylon graft.[43]

The author's first carotid endarterectomy was performed on April 16, 1957.[44] With increasing experience, the various procedures described above were abandoned, with the exception of endarterectomy, which has

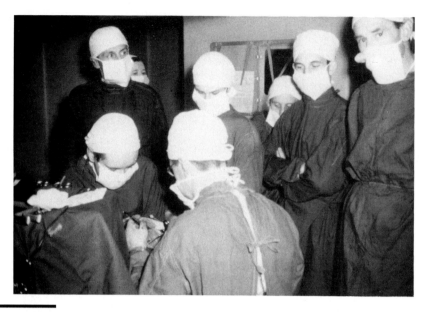

FIGURE 3.

Photograph taken at St. Mary's Hospital May 19, 1954, of the historic carotid reconstruction operation. Mr. Eastcott (back to camera) is seated, operating. Professor Rob is standing, on the far right. (Courtesy of Dr. George R. Dunlop.)

become the standard operation. Table 1 lists in chronologic order the early procedures performed for the treatment of extracranial cerebrovascular disease.

The case described by Cooley and colleagues is of interest in that an external shunt was used for cerebral protection, the first reported use of a shunt for carotid endarterectomy. The shunt consisted of a polyvinyl tube with a 14-gauge needle at its lower end and a 16-gauge needle at its upper or internal carotid end. Additional cerebral protection was attempted by immersing the patient's head in crushed ice for 30 minutes. In spite of this, the patient suffered an operation-related stroke from which he recovered rapidly over the course of several weeks.[47]

I first used an external shunt similar to Cooley's, using 13-gauge needles, on January 6, 1958, with no problems, and continued to use the external shunt selectively until October 14, 1960, when I first used an intraluminal inlying shunt, at the suggestion of E. Stanley Crawford. I have continued to use the inlying shunt first selectively and then routinely since that time. The early experience with this type of shunt was described in the literature in 1962.[48]

A fascinating aspect of this subject is a study of famous people who have had strokes. Marccello Malpighi, one of the great early microscopists, suffered his first stroke at age 66 years, on July 25, 1694, and died of another "apoplexy" on November 29, 1694.[6, 49]

Louis Pasteur had a series of transient ischemic attacks affecting largely his speech area, but also his left side over a period of some 10 years before he finally died September 28, 1895, at the age of 73 years.[6, 49]

Several intriguing reports have speculated on the fate of nations as

TABLE 1.

The First Carotid Reconstructions for Cerebrovascular Insufficiency, Listed in Chronologic Order

Author	Date of Operation	Degree of Stenosis	Procedure	Restoration of Flow
Carrea et al.[38]	10/20/51	Partial	End-to-end anastomosis external carotid to internal carotid	Yes
Strully et al.[39]	1/28/53	Total	Thromboendarterectomy followed by ligation and resection	No
DeBakey[40]	8/7/53	Total	Thromboendarterectomy	Yes
Eastcott et al.[41]	5/19/54; 6/54	Both partial	End-to-end anastomosis common carotid to internal carotid; thromboendarterectomy	Yes Yes
Denman et al.[45]	7/14/54	Total	Resection with homograft	Yes
Lin et al.[46]	12/55	Partial	Resection with saphenous vein graft	Yes
Murphey and Miller[42]	2/6/56; 2/24/56	Total; partial	Thromboendarterectomies	Yes
Cooley et al.[47]	3/8/56	Partial	Endarterectomy	Yes
Lyons and Galbraith[43]	8/9/56	Partial	Subclavian-carotid nylon bypass graft	Yes

affected by strokes occurring in their leaders. One world-famous figure who suffered from and eventually died of cerebrovascular deterioration was Marshal Paul von Hindenburg. Certainly, his action in authorizing Hitler to form a cabinet in 1933 was a decision that altered the course of history. Whether anyone could have stopped Hitler at this time is subject to speculation, but in his senile and demented state, von Hindenburg refused or was unable to involve himself in trouble or controversy. He was so far gone mentally that his Secretary of State actually had to write down for him word for word the questions put to any caller.[50]

In Russia, V. I. Lenin also suffered from cerebrovascular troubles. He experienced several transient ischemic episodes, finally had a complete right hemiplegia, and died of his third stroke at the early age of 54 years on January 21, 1924. Prior to his illness, Lenin had been responsible for elevating Josef Stalin to several important positions in the government, but in the last years of his life, he had grave doubts about Stalin and wanted Leon Trotsky to assume the more important posts. Had Lenin lived to make Trotsky his heir apparent instead of Stalin, who knows what the course of modern history might have been.[6, 50]

Ironically, Josef Stalin, the Soviet dictator who succeeded Lenin, died of a stroke at age 73 years on March 5, 1953, the cerebrovascular accident having occurred 4 days earlier on March 1, 1953.[6]

In our own country, no less than ten American presidents have suffered from or died of cerebrovascular disease. These include John Quincy Adams, John Tyler, Millard Fillmore, Chester Arthur, Andrew Johnson, Woodrow Wilson, Franklin Delano Roosevelt, Dwight D. Eisenhower, and possibly Rutherford B. Hayes, William Howard Taft, and Warren G. Harding.[6, 51, 52]

A very dramatic example is the case of Woodrow Wilson. He had a stroke in September of 1919, with paralysis of his left arm and leg, which improved to some degree; but in October, he suffered another episode. Again, he improved, but was almost totally incapacitated. Although unable to carry out the duties of the presidency, he nevertheless did not step down from office. His term ended on March 4, 1921, when he was succeeded by Warren G. Harding. Woodrow Wilson died February 3, 1924 of a massive cerebral infarction. It has been stated by those who have studied the President's illness in detail that Wilson's cerebrovascular disease significantly contributed to the defeat of the United States' support for the League of Nations.[6, 50, 51]

The illness of Franklin Delano Roosevelt is well known. In 1943, he reportedly had severe symptoms of cerebrovascular insufficiency with multiple ischemic episodes. How this disease affected the Yalta agreements of 1945 and the subsequent Cold War is a matter of speculation. His sudden death at the Georgia Warm Springs on April 12, 1945 was said to be due to a massive cerebral hemorrhage, but no autopsy was performed.[6, 51, 52]

The most recent cerebrovascular episodes in a chief executive were experienced by Dwight D. Eisenhower. His "little strokes" were said to be due to intracranial disease. His death came ultimately, however, from complications of heart disease rather than stroke.

In contrast to the individuals listed above, the late Mayor Richard Daley of Chicago, after having transient cerebral ischemia, was subjected to carotid endarterectomy by Hushang Javid in April of 1974, with complete success and restoration of brain function to normal.

In cerebrovascular insufficiency, *morbidity* at times may be more important than mortality. Thus, the *quality* of survival is emphasized as a feature of this disease, more so perhaps than in coronary artery disease, and underlines the main role of carotid endarterectomy as one of stroke prevention.[53]

The surgeon's role in the treatment of cerebral ischemic syndromes by means of carotid endarterectomy has been substantiated by the recent reports of the results of two large randomized trials, the North American Symptomatic Carotid Endarterectomy Trial[54] and the Medical Research Council European Carotid Surgery Trial,[55] demonstrating the efficacy of surgery in preventing strokes.

In the last 40 years, there has been a widespread renewal of interest in strokes. All aspects of the field have been reexamined, including the role of the surgeon, and the interest continues unabated.

ACKNOWLEDGMENT

I am indebted to Leslie W. Ottinger, M.D. for providing me with material on David Fleming and Amos Twitchell.

REFERENCES

1. Thompson JE: The development of carotid artery surgery. *Arch Surg* 1973; 107:643–648.
2. Thompson JE, Patman RD, Talkington CM: Carotid surgery for cerebrovascular insufficiency. *Curr Probl Surg* 1978; 15:1–68.
3. Dandy WE: *Surgery of the Brain*. Hagerstown, WF Prior, 1945.
4. Paré A: *The Workes of That Famous Chirurgion Ambrose Parey. Translated Out of Latine and Compared With the French*, 4th English ed. London, 1678. (Reprinted, New York, Milford House, 1968.)
5. Gurdjian ES, Gurdjian ES: History of occlusive cerebrovascular disease. From Wepfer to Moniz. *Arch Neurol* 1979; 36:340–343.
6. Fields WS, Lemak NA: *A History of Stroke*. New York, Oxford University Press, 1989.
7. Cutter IS: Ligation of the common carotid—Amos Twitchell. *Surg Gynecol Obstet Int Abst Surg* 1929; 48:1–3.
8. Petit JL: *Chirug Mem de l'Acad Roy des Sciences*. Paris, Royal Academy of Science, 1765.
9. Hebenstreit EBG: *Zusatze zu Benj. Bell's Abhandlung von den Geschwuren and deren Behandlung*. Germany, 1793.
10. Wood JR: Early history of the operation of ligature of the primitive carotid artery. *N Y J Med* 1857; July:1–59.
11. Abernethy J: Surgical observations. *Surgical Works* 1804; 2:193–209.
12. Hamby WB: *Intracranial Aneurysms*. Springfield, Charles C Thomas, 1952.
13. Coley RW: Case of rupture of the carotid artery, and wounds of several of its branches, successfully treated by tying the common trunk of the carotid itself. *Med Chir J Rev* 1817; 3:1–4.
14. Keevil JJ: David Fleming and the operation for ligation of the carotid artery. *Br J Surg* 1949; 37:92–95.
15. Cogswell MF: Account of an operation for the extirpation of a tumour, in which a ligature was applied to the carotid artery. *N Engl J Med Surg* 1824; 13:357–360.
16. Twitchell A: Gun-shot wound of the face and neck. Ligature of the carotid artery. *N Engl Q J Med Surg* 1842; 1:188–193.
17. Cooper A: Second case of carotid aneurysm. *Med Chir Trans* 1809; 1:222–233.
18. Cooper A: Account of the first successful operation performed on the common carotid artery for aneurysm in the year 1808 with the postmortem examination in the year 1821. *Guys Hosp Rep* 1836; 1:53–59.
19. Wyeth JA: Prize essay. Essays upon the surgical anatomy and history of the common, external and internal carotid arteries and the surgical anatomy of the innominate and subclavian arteries. *Appendix to Transactions of the AMA* 1878; 29:1–245.
20. Osler W: *The Principles and Practice of Medicine*, 7th ed. New York, D Appleton, 1909.
21. Heberden W: Epilepsy, head-ache, palsy and apoplexy, and St. Vitus dance,

in *Commentaries on the History and Cure of Diseases*. London, T Payne, 1802.

22. Gull WW: Case of occlusion of the innominate and left carotid. *Guys Hosp Rep* 1855; 1:12.

23. Savory WS: Case of a young woman in whom the main arteries of both upper extremities and of the left side of the neck were throughout completely obliterated. *Med Chir Trans* 1856; 39:205–219.

24. Broadbent WH: Absence of pulsations on both radial arteries, vessels being full of blood. *Trans Clin Soc* 1875; 8:165–168.

25. Penzoldt F: Uber thrombose (autochtone oder embolische) der carotis. *Deutsches Arch f Klin Med* 1881; 28:80–93.

26. Chiari H: Uber des verhalten des teilungswinkels der carotis communis bei der endarteritis chronica deformans. *Verh Dtsch Ges Pathol* 1905; 9:326–330.

27. Hunt JR: The role of the carotid arteries in the causation of vascular lesions of the brain, with remarks on certain special features of the symptomatology. *Am J Med Sci* 1914; 147:704–713.

28. Móniz E: L'encephalographic arterielle son importance dan la localization des tumeurs cerebrales. *Rev Neurol (Paris)* 1927; 2:72–90.

29. Sjöqvist O: Uber intrakranielle aneurysmen der arteria carotis und deren beziehung zur ophthalmoplegischen migraine. *Nervenarzt* 1936; 9:233–241.

30. Móniz E, Lima A, de Lacerda R: Hemiplegies par thrombose de la carotide interne. *Presse Med* 1937; 45:977–980.

31. Chao WH, Kwan ST, Lyman RS, et al: Thrombosis of the left internal carotid artery. *Arch Surg* 1938; 37:100–111.

32. Johnson HC, Walker AE: The angiographic diagnosis of spontaneous thrombosis of the internal and common carotid arteries. *J Neurosurg* 1951; 8:631–659.

33. Fisher M: Occlusion of the internal carotid artery. *Arch Neurol Psychiatry* 1951; 65:346–377.

34. Fisher M: Occlusion of the carotid arteries. *Arch Neurol Psychiatry* 1954; 72:187–204.

35. Thompson JE: *Surgery for Cerebrovascular Insufficiency (Stroke)*. Springfield, Charles C Thomas, 1968.

36. Gurdjian ES, Webster JE: Stroke resulting from internal carotid artery thrombosis in the neck. *JAMA* 1953; 151:541–545.

37. Wylie EJ, Kerr E, Davies O: Experimental and clinical experiences with use of fascia lata applied as a graft about major arteries after thromboendarterectomy and aneurysmorrhaphy. *Surg Gynecol Obstet* 1951; 93:257–272.

38. Carrea R, Molins M, Murphy G: Surgical treatment of spontaneous thrombosis of the internal carotid artery in the neck. Carotid-carotideal anastomosis. Report of a case. *Acta Neurol Latin Am* 1955; 1:71–78.

39. Strully KJ, Hurwitt ES, Blankenberg HW: Thromboendarterectomy for thrombosis of the internal carotid artery in the neck. *J Neurosurg* 1953; 10:474–482.

40. DeBakey ME: Successful carotid endarterectomy for cerebrovascular insufficiency. *JAMA* 1975; 233:1083–1085.

41. Eastcott HHG, Pickering GW, Rob CG: Reconstruction of internal carotid artery in a patient with intermittent attacks of hemiplegia. *Lancet* 1954; 2:994–996.

42. Murphey F, Miller JH: Carotid insufficiency—diagnosis and surgical treatment. *J Neurosurg* 1959; 16:1–23.

43. Lyons C, Galbraith JG: Surgical treatment of atherosclerotic occlusion of the internal carotid artery. *Ann Surg* 1957; 146:487–496.

44. Thompson JE, Austin DJ, Patman RD: Carotid endarterectomy for cerebrovascular insufficiency: Long term results in 592 patients followed up to thirteen years. *Ann Surg* 1970; 172:663–679.

45. Denman FR, Ehni G, Duty WS: Insidious thrombotic occlusion of cervical arteries treated by arterial graft, a case report. *Surgery* 1955; 38:569–577.

46. Lin PM, Javid H, Doyle EJ: Partial internal carotid artery occlusion treated by primary resection and vein graft. *J Neurosurg* 1956; 13:650–655.

47. Cooley DA, Al-Naaman YD, Carton CA: Surgical treatment of arteriosclerotic occlusion of common carotid artery. *J Neurosurg* 1956; 13:500–506.

48. Thompson JE, Austin DJ: Surgical treatment of arteriosclerotic occlusions of the carotid artery in the neck. *Surgery* 1962; 51:74–83.

49. Fishbein M: Strokes 1. Some literary descriptions. *Postgrad Med* 1965; 37:194–198.

50. Friedlander WJ: About three old men: An inquiry into how cerebral arteriosclerosis has altered world politics. *Stroke* 1972; 3:467–473.

51. Fishbein M: Strokes 2. American presidents who had strokes. *Postgrad Med* 1965; 37:200–208.

52. Robertson CW: Some observations on presidential illnesses. *Boston Med Q* 1957; 8:33–43.

53. Thompson JE: Carotid endarterectomy, 1982—the state of the art. 1983; 70:371–376.

54. North American Symptomatic Carotid Endarterectomy Trial Collaborators: Beneficial effect of carotid endarterectomy in symptomatic patients with high-grade carotid stenosis. *N Engl J Med* 1991; 325:445–453.

55. European Carotid Surgery Trialists' Collaborative Group: MRC European Carotid Surgery Trial: Interim results for symptomatic patients with severe (70–99%) or with mild (0–29%) stenosis. *Lancet* 1991; 337:1235–1243.

Symptomatic Carotid Artery Disease

D. EUGENE STRANDNESS, JR., M.D.

Atherosclerosis of the carotid bifurcation and its relationship to ischemic cerebrovascular events has an interesting history. Although coronary artery disease and occlusive lesions of the peripheral arteries long have been recognized as a cause of ischemia, it took a great deal of time before the association of carotid artery disease and stroke was accepted and acknowledged widely. As Friedman points out, it was Ramsey Hunt in 1913 who played a role in bringing this fact to the attention of physicians. He wrote, ". . . I would urge that in all cases presenting cerebral symptoms of vascular origin, that the main arteries of the neck be carefully examined for a possible diminution or absence of pulsation. Obstructive lesions of these vessels are overlooked from failure to make clinical and pathological examination from this point of view."[1] By 1927, Moniz had developed cerebral arteriography. The evolution of this method permitted the recognition of carotid artery disease as a possible contributor to the cause of stroke. It took until 1951, however, for C. Miller Fisher to point out that most strokes clearly were of embolic origin.[2] He stated, "It was logical to look more proximally, namely in the internal carotid artery, for unrecognized disease."

When the relationship between disease of the carotid artery and stroke was appreciated, it was very soon thereafter that attempts were made to correct the problem surgically. Several surgeons must be given credit for approaching this problem during this time frame. Those who performed procedures on the carotid artery include Carrea, Molins, and Murphy from Argentina, who anastomosed the external carotid to the distal internal carotid artery.[3] In 1953, Strully, Hurwitt, and Blankenberg attempted the first thromboendarterectomy of the carotid artery.[4] DeBakey in 1953 performed one of the first successful endarterectomies of the carotid bulb.[5] There is little doubt that the procedure done by Eastcott, Pickering, and Rob in 1954 is the one most remembered and quoted.[6] This report is thought to have provided the impetus for surgeons to begin a more aggressive surgical approach to the correction of carotid bifurcation stenosis.

The number of carotid endarterectomies being done escalated gradually until the mid-1980s, when, in terms of total numbers, this procedure was second only to coronary bypass grafting. In 1985, 107,000 carotid endarterectomies were performed in hospitals in the United States (other than Veterans Administration hospitals).[7] It was about this time that

Advances in Vascular Surgery, vol. 1.
©1993, Mosby–Year Book, Inc.

many in the neurology community began to take issue with the role of the operation. It may have been the report by Easton and Sherman in 1977 that sparked the concern.[8] This study showed that, in Springfield, Illinois, the combined morbidity and mortality rate from carotid endarterectomy was 20%!

Given these data and the concern that the results with carotid endarterectomy might not be any better than those obtainable with medical therapy, the operation came under greater scrutiny than any other procedure that vascular surgeons perform.[9, 10] There was a joint cooperative study of carotid endarterectomy carried out in the 1960s, but the results of this trial were inconclusive because of the high rate of perioperative stroke and death (11%).[11] Because so many questions remained unanswered, demands were made for multicenter, randomized clinical trials of carotid endarterectomy compared with aspirin and conventional medical therapy.

It must be remembered that the controversies centered around two major concerns: the safety of the operation and its efficacy in the prevention of stroke. Although there was no doubt that the early published results with regard to endarterectomy were less than optimal, it was clear that, with more experience, surgical technique improved and rates of stroke and death associated with the operation decreased. In fact, numerous reports show that the combined morbidity and mortality rate from the procedure can be kept below 5%. Interestingly, these reports were discounted by the neurology community because the reported series were not prospective, not randomized, and not reported by neurologists.

With regard to the efficacy of carotid endarterectomy, how effective is the procedure in preventing stroke? It was estimated, based on historic data, that the incidence of stroke after a transient ischemic attack (TIA) was 5% per year for the first 3 years and 3% per year thereafter. As will be shown later, this underestimated the outcome for the medically treated patients in both the North American Symptomatic Carotid Endarterectomy Trial (NASCET) and the European Carotid Surgery Trial (ECST).[12, 13]

Two other issues are of concern to surgeons who work in this field. First, TIAs were not considered by neurologists to be adverse events, since they did not result in irreversible neurologic damage. Yet, a TIA was considered an acceptable inclusion criterion for entry into a clinical trial, but repeat TIA was not considered a therapeutic failure! The second issue relates to internal carotid occlusion.

If atherosclerosis progresses to occlusion of the internal carotid artery, this is an adverse outcome.[14–16] The development of an occlusion is not considered by neurologists to be an event, however, unless it is accompanied by a stroke. This makes little sense to me, since the therapy failed to halt the progression of the disease. From a surgical standpoint, a perioperative occlusion of the internal carotid artery is a complication of the procedure whether or not the patient has a neurologic event. This same consideration should be applied to nonsurgical forms of therapy.

All of the above issues are very important when considering the role of carotid endarterectomy for the treatment of carotid artery disease. They are equally important in the asymptomatic patient. This subset of patients will be dealt with in a separate chapter in this volume.

PROSPECTIVE STUDIES

The two major prospective studies mounted in the 1980s to evaluate the role of endarterectomy in symptomatic patients were the NASCET and the ECST.[12, 13] Both trials were designed to test carotid endarterectomy against conventional medical therapy for control of symptomatic carotid artery disease. Conventional medical therapy was defined as control and treatment of those risk factors thought to be of importance in the pathogenesis of atherosclerosis of the carotid artery and their contribution to the development of ischemic cerebrovascular events. The only drug in use that was thought to influence the lesion directly at the carotid bifurcation was aspirin. The effectiveness of aspirin for the prevention of strokes was suggested by combining the results of many clinical trials (meta-analysis).[17]

The entry criteria for the trials were similar in that patients had to have had a hemispheric TIA, monocular blindness lasting less than 24 hours, or a nondisabling stroke. The event had to have taken place within the previous 120 days. All patients under the age of 80 years who qualified for entry into the trial underwent selective carotid arteriography. The estimate of the degree of diameter reduction was based on the dimensions at the site of narrowing compared with the diameter of the internal carotid artery beyond the bulb. To qualify for randomization in the NASCET, the degree of diameter reduction had to be in the range of 30% to 99%. Lesser degrees of stenosis were permitted for entry into the ECST.

The qualifying criteria for entry into the NASCET and the ECST were similar, but selection for randomization was not the same. In the ECST, the patient would be entered only if the neurologist and surgeon were "substantially uncertain" whether to recommend carotid endarterectomy for the patient. If both agreed that surgery was indicated, the patient was not randomized. No such decision making was permitted in the NASCET.

In the NASCET, all patients (medical and surgical) were prescribed aspirin, 325 mg three times a day. It was interesting that, at the time of consideration for entry into the trial, 89% of the patients already were taking aspirin. This fact, in and of itself, might have represented a failure of antiplatelet therapy, at least, of aspirin. In the ECST, it is not clear how many patients actually were given aspirin. The only statement in the report concerning this issue is as follows: "Clinicians were asked to ensure that patients in the two groups received similar and appropriate treatment: this usually included aspirin, . . ."[13] Thus, it is not certain how many patients in the ECST actually received an antiplatelet agent during the course of the study.

The NASCET had been in operation for only 3 years when the stopping rule had to be invoked. It became clear that patients with 70% to 99% stenosis were treated best by endarterectomy and not by conventional medical therapy. When this fact was noted, the National Institute of Neurological Disease and Stroke issued a clinical alert to the physicians of the United States bringing this finding to their attention. At the same time, the interim results of the ECST were made known and, as will be discussed, the outcome in that trial was very similar to the outcome noted by the NASCET.

TRIAL DESIGN

In the NASCET, 50 centers participated throughout the United States and Canada. In each center, there was a participating vascular surgeon or neurosurgeon and a neurologist. To qualify as a center, evidence had to be provided that the perioperative morbidity and mortality for carotid endarterectomy at the site was less than 5%. In the ECST, 80 centers from 14 countries participated. For the surgical therapy, the postoperative period was 30 days. For the medically treated patients, 2 days were added, since this was the median time to randomization. These periods proved to be of interest in terms of the strokes that took place during this time.

In the NASCET, surgery was done promptly after randomization. A similar policy was suggested for the ECST, but operation could be delayed for 4 to 6 weeks if a recent stroke had occurred. The accepted events for inclusion in the study were hemispheric TIA or stroke. Patients with a stroke had to be able to function independently in order to qualify for entry into the trials. The average duration of follow-up was 18 months for the NASCET and 3 years for the ECST.

OUTCOME

The early event rate—30 days for surgery and 32 days for medical therapy—obviously is of great importance. In the NASCET, the combined perioperative and postoperative morbidity and mortality rate was 5.8%. When the analysis was confined to major events (major stroke and death), the rate was 2.1%. The surgical mortality rate was 0.6%. The medically treated patients had a stroke rate of 3.3% and a mortality rate of 0.3% for the first 32 days after randomization. Thus, the timing of therapy after a TIA or stroke is of great importance.

In the ECST, the perioperative and postoperative event rate was not as good. During the first 30 days after operation, the stroke or death rate was 7.5%.

For the 328 patients randomized to surgery in the NASCET, the cumulative risk of stroke at 2 years was 9%. For the medically treated patients, the cumulative risk of stroke was 26%. This represented an absolute risk reduction of 17% $\pm$ 3.5% ($P < .001$). For major or fatal ipsilateral stroke, the cumulative risk for the surgically treated patients was 2.5% compared to 13.1% for the medically treated patients. This represented an absolute risk reduction of 10.6% $\pm$ 2.5% ($P < .001$; Table 1).

In the ECST, for the 778 patients with greater than 70% stenosis and a mean follow-up period of 3 years, the risk of stroke, death, surgically related stroke and death, and ipsilateral stroke was 12.3% for those treated surgically and 21.9% for those treated medically ($P < .01$).

The ECST did come to the conclusion that, for lesions with stenosis in the range of 0% to 30%, the event rate was so low for the medically treated patients that it was unlikely that any benefit might accrue from

TABLE 1.

Adverse Events at 2 Years of Follow-up in the North American Symptomatic Carotid Endarterectomy Trial

Event	Number of Medical Patients* (%)	Number of Surgical Patients† (%)	Relative Risk Reduction (%)
Any ipsilateral stroke	61 (26)	26 (9)‡	65
Any stroke	64 (28)	34 (13)‡	54
Any stroke or death	73 (32)	41 (16)‡	51
Major or fatal ipsilateral stroke	29 (13)	8 (3)‡	81
Any major or fatal stroke	29 (13)	10 (4)‡	72
Any major stroke or death	38 (18)	19 (8)§	56

*N = 331.
†N = 328
‡$P < .001$.
§$P < .01$.

surgery in these individuals. Recruitment for such patients was discontinued.

In both the NASCET and the ECST, the data with regard to stenoses in the range of 30% to 69% were not sufficiently clear to demonstrate the effectiveness of operation. Recruitment is continuing for this category of patients in both trials.

DISCUSSION

It appears that we have reached an important milestone in the treatment of carotid artery disease. Given the interim results of these two trials, it is certain now that carotid endarterectomy is more effective than conventional therapy in symptomatic patients with stenoses in the range of 70% to 99%. It also appears that the gradient of risk increases as the degree of stenosis increases, even in this quite narrow range, that is, stenosis of 90% to 99% is more dangerous than is stenosis of 70% to 79%.

Another important fact to emerge from these studies was the lack of comorbid risk factors found during analysis of the data, suggesting that medical therapy would be better than surgical therapy under any circumstances. This is very important for the surgeon, whose major consideration is estimating "surgical risk" in the classic sense and not in terms of whether there are factors other than the carotid bifurcation lesion itself that should dictate the approach to therapy.

The positive results of these two clinical trials have generated several important questions. Given the fact that the patients were followed closely, natural history data on the fate of the lesions should be available. For example, in the medical arm of the trial, it would be very interesting to know what actually occurred at the bifurcation that led to a stroke. Was it progression to total occlusion of the internal carotid or were other factors involved? Likewise, in the surgical arm of the trial, there is no information on the status of the operated segment. Although we know the stroke rate, we do not know the incidence of perioperative, postoperative, and late occlusion of the internal carotid artery. This type of information is of great interest and importance to both surgeons and other physicians because it helps to clarify the etiology of perioperative stroke and the durability of the operation. The fact that such data are not available is a serious limitation of these trials.

Questions already have been raised as to what the results of these trials will mean to our daily practice. For example, what if a patient presents with a TIA or stroke but is found by arteriography to have 50% or 60% carotid stenosis? This raises several questions and possible controversies. Should operation be withheld because the lesion does not quite reach the stage of a 70% diameter reduction? The method used to determine the degree of diameter reduction in the NASCET was measurement of the internal carotid artery distal to the bulb for use as the normal reference vessel. By this method, 50% reduction in vessel diameter at the level of the carotid bulb would represent 0% stenosis. In addition, this method of measurement is subject to wide discrepancy,[18] depending on the type of arteriogram employed, the number of views taken, and the interrater variability that can be expected in interpretation of the arteriograms. There are no hard and fast rules but (in general, a variability of ±20%) in estimating the diameter reduction is not unreasonable.

Several other problems will undoubtedly surface as we take a new look at the role of endarterectomy. What about the patient with an occluded internal carotid artery on one side, 50% stenosis of the contralateral artery, and a TIA? Will the surgeon be forced to rigidly follow the guidelines of the trials? One would hope that common sense and good judgment would prevail under these circumstances.

There are no firm guidelines to follow, and decisions regarding therapy will depend on many factors, not the least of which is the personal experience of individual surgeons. The issue will be surgical competence. The NASCET and ECST results provide firm guidelines in regard to appropriate expectations for stroke reduction from carotid endarterectomy. Clearly if a surgeon's morbidity and mortality rate from the procedure begins to exceed that of medically treated patients, both short- and long-term benefits of the operation will be lost. Can we determine a satisfactory range of surgical morbidity and mortality rates that are pertinent to clinical presentation and indications for the procedure? The guidelines published by an ad hoc committee of the American Heart Association provide a starting point.[19] The acceptable combined morbidity and mortality rate should be as follows: less than 3% for asymptomatic patients, less than 5% for patients with TIAs, less than 7% for patients with stroke, and less than 10% for patients undergoing repeat procedures. These results should be easy for experienced surgeons to attain. In fact, better results are common in many published series.

Finally, potentially important savings can be accrued if proper screening procedures are carried out when patients first come to medical attention. Patients should first be studied by ultrasonic duplex scanning to determine the status of the carotid bulb.[20] If the bulb is normal or has only minimal disease, there is little need to proceed with arteriography because surgical therapy will not be considered. This policy will reduce the cost to the health care system as well as minimize the number of complications from the angiographic procedure.

REFERENCES

1. Friedman SG: Operation on the carotid artery, in Freidman SG (ed): *A History of Vascular Surgery*. Mount Kisco, NY, Futura, 1989, p 157–171.
2. Fischer CM: Occlusion of the internal carotid artery. *Arch Neurol Psychiatry* 1951; 65:346–377.
3. Carrea R, Molins M, Murphy G: Surgical treatment of spontaneous thrombosis of the internal carotid artery in the neck. Carotid-carotideal anastomosis. *Acta Neurol Latinoamer* 1955; 1:71–78.
4. Strully KJ, Hurwitt ES, Blankenberg HW: Thrombo-endarterectomy for thrombosis of the internal carotid artery in the neck. *J Neurosurg* 1953; 10:474–462.
5. DeBakey ME: Successful carotid endarterectomy for cerebrovascular insufficiency. Nineteen year followup. *JAMA* 1975; 233:1083–1085.
6. Eastcott HHG, Pickering GW, Rob C: Reconstruction of internal carotid artery in a patient with intermittent attacks of hemiplegia. *Lancet* 1954; 2:994–996.
7. Pokras R, Dyken ML: Dramatic changes in the performance of endarterectomy for diseases of the extracranial arteries of the head. *Stroke* 1988; 10:1289–1290.
8. Easton JD, Sherman DG: Stroke and mortality rate in carotid endarterectomy. 228 consecutive operations. *Stroke* 1977; 8:565–568.
9. Barnett HJM, Plum F, Walton JN: Carotid endarterectomy: An expression of concern. *Stroke* 1984; 15:941–943.
10. Chambers BR, Norris JW: The case against surgery for asymptomatic carotid stenosis. *Stroke* 1984; 15:964–967.
11. Fields WS, Maslenikov V, Meyer IS, et al: Joint study of extracranial artery occlusion V. Progress report of prognosis following surgery or nonsurgical treatment for transient cerebral ischemic attacks and cervical carotid arterial lesions. *JAMA* 1970; 211:1993–2003.
12. North American Symptomatic Carotid Endarterectomy Trial Collaborators: Beneficial effect of carotid endarterectomy in symptomatic patients with high-grade carotid stenosis. *N Engl J Med* 1991; 325:445–463.
13. European Carotid Surgery Trialists' Collaborative Group: MRC European Carotid Surgery Trial. Interim results for symptomatic patients with severe (70–99%) or with mild (0–29%) stenosis. *Lancet* 1991; 337:1235–1243.
14. Nicholls SC, Kohler TR, Bergelin RO, et al: Carotid artery occlusion, natural history. *J Vasc Surg* 1986; 4:479–485.
15. Nicholls SC, Bergelin RO, Strandness DE Jr: Neurological sequelae of unilateral carotid artery occlusion. Immediate and late. *J Vasc Surg* 1989; 10:542–548.
16. Cote R, Barnett HJM, Taylor DM: Internal carotid artery occlusion. A prospective study. *Stroke* 1983; 14:898–902.
17. Antiplatelet Trialists Collaboration: Secondary prevention of vascular disease by prolonged antiplatelet treatment. *BMJ* 1988; 296:320–331.
18. Chikos PM, Fisher LD, Hirsch JH, et al: Observer variability in evaluating extracranial arterial stenosis. *Stroke* 1983; 14:885–892.
19. Beebe HG, Clagett GP, DeWeese JA, et al: Assessing risk associated with ca-

rotid endarterectomy: A statement for health professionals by an ad hoc committee on carotid surgery standards of the stroke council, American Heart Association. *Stroke* 1989; 20:314–315.

20. Langlois YE, Roederer GO, Strandness DE Jr: Ultrasonic evaluation of the carotid bifurcation. *Echocardiography* 1987; 4:141–159.

Treatment of Asymptomatic Carotid Stenosis

ROBERT W. HOBSON II, M.D.

Cerebrovascular disease is the third leading cause of death in the western world, accounting for 9% of all deaths in the United States, and it remains a major cause of disability among the elderly population. About 450,000 new strokes occur each year in this country, and nearly 75% result from thromboembolic disease. Although the efficacy of carotid endarterectomy in patients with a transient ischemic attack (TIA) or nondisabling stroke and ipsilateral carotid stenosis of 70% or greater has been confirmed by prospective, randomized, clinical trials,[1-3] controversy continues regarding the indications for intervention in patients with asymptomatic carotid stenosis. If all strokes were preceded by a TIA, as has been reported by some authors,[4, 5] a decision to await the development of a TIA before performing carotid endarterectomy in patients with asymptomatic stenosis would seem appropriate. Follow-up population studies, however, have demonstrated that substantially higher percentages of patients who sustain a stroke do not experience a preceding TIA. In one recently published, prospective, randomized trial on asymptomatic carotid stenosis,[6] 50% of patients had a stroke without antecedent TIA. Of additional concern is the question of whether TIA prevention should be included in the therapeutic considerations regarding the efficacy of endarterectomy in patients with asymptomatic stenosis. Clearly, preventing minor neurologic deficits that last no more than several minutes does not seem to jus-

TABLE 1.

Annual Percentage Rate of Vascular Events Over Period of Follow-up*

Degree of Stenosis	TIA†	Stroke	Cardiac	Vascular Death
<50% (mild)	1.0	1.3	2.7	1.8
50% to 75% (moderate)	3.0	1.3	6.6	3.3
>75% (severe)	7.2	3.3	8.3	6.5

*From Norris JW, Zhu CZ, Bornstein NM, et al: *Stroke* 1991; 22:485. Used by permission.
†TIA = transient ischemic attack.

Advances in Vascular Surgery, vol. 1.
©1993, Mosby–Year Book, Inc.

tify such a consideration. Because TIAs are established precursors of stroke, however, with an annual incidence of cerebral infarction despite optimal medical (including antiplatelet medication) management,[1] preventing TIAs may be as important as preventing nondisabling strokes.[7, 8]

DEFINING TERMINOLOGY

An asymptomatic carotid bruit is associated with minimal risk of stroke, as defined in population-based studies.[9, 10] Recognizing that a bruit occurs with stenoses as minimal as 20% to 30%, Norris and colleagues[11] have confirmed that, within a group of patients with lesser stenoses, the annual rate of stroke is minimal. As the area-reducing stenosis increases from 50% to 75% and then to greater than 75%, however, the incidence of TIA and stroke increase significantly (Table 1).

Consequently, a shift in emphasis toward diagnosing severe and hemodynamically significant asymptomatic carotid stenosis has occurred during recent years. The severity of stenosis has been defined arterio-

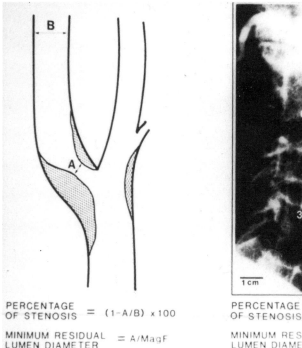

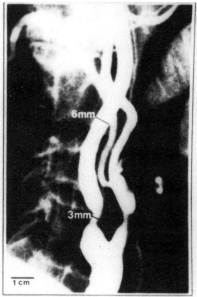

PERCENTAGE OF STENOSIS $= (1 - A/B) \times 100$

MINIMUM RESIDUAL LUMEN DIAMETER $= A/MagF$

PERCENTAGE OF STENOSIS $= (1 - 3/6) \times 100 = 50\%$

MINIMUM RESIDUAL LUMEN DIAMETER $= 3/1.4 = 2.2$

FIGURE 1.

The percentage of stenosis is calculated by dividing the least transverse diameter of the internal carotid artery at the stenosis (A) by the diameter of the distal, uninvolved artery (B). The minimum residual lumen diameter is equivalent to the least transverse diameter (A) divided by the magnification factor *(MagF)* of the arteriogram. The example *(right)* illustrates a 50% stenosis by diameter and a minimum residual lumen diameter of 2.2 (From Lynch TG, Hobson RW: Noninvasive cerebrovascular diagnostic techniques, in Wilson SE, Veith FJ, Hobson RW, et al (eds): *Vascular Surgery: Principles and Practice.* New York, McGraw Hill, 1987, pp 105–134. Used by permission.)

graphically as a 50% reduction in luminal diameter of the artery or a calculated 75% reduction in its cross-sectional area (Fig 1). The percentage of stenosis is determined by comparing the least transverse diameter at the stenosis with the diameter of the postbulbar internal carotid artery once its walls become parallel. Coupled with positive results of noninvasive studies such as ocular pneumoplethysmography (Gee-OPG) [12] or duplex scanning,[13] a 50% diameter stenosis or 75% area-reducing stenosis is a threshold lesion for considering surgical intervention in asymptomatic patients.

SURGICAL CONSIDERATIONS

Several assumptions have been presented previously and now are confirmed by review of the literature regarding the efficacy of carotid endarterectomy in patients with asymptomatic carotid stenosis. Patients with high-grade carotid stenosis can be identified accurately from the pool of patients with cervical bruits by noninvasive techniques,[12, 13] and arteriographic confirmation can be obtained at little risk.[6, 14] In addition, the assumption that TIA and nondisabling stroke represent a clinical continuum,[15] which is accompanied in some individuals by positive findings on computed tomography, has become accepted more widely. Silent or asymptomatic infarcts also have been observed on computed tomographic scans of the brain. In the Toronto study,[16] symptomatic patients with TIA and with or without carotid stenosis were compared to patients with asymptomatic carotid stenosis. Silent infarcts were seen in 19% of the asymptomatic group compared with 30% of the patients with TIA and no carotid stenosis and 47% of the patients with TIA and carotid stenosis. All infarcts were lacunar in size. Finally, carotid endarterectomy can be performed with low perioperative complication rates (Table 2).

Surgeons encounter patients with asymptomatic carotid stenosis under three different clinical circumstances: referral because of cervical bruit in the absence of lateralizing neurologic symptoms; the presence of

TABLE 2.

Morbidity and Mortality Associated With Carotid Endarterectomy for Asymptomatic Carotid Disease in Different Studies

Authors	Operations	Mortality	Morbidity	
			Transient	Permanent
Thompson et al.[17]	167	0	2(1.2%)	2(1.2%)
Moore et al.[18]	78	0	2(2.6%)	0
Hertzer et al.[19]	95	1(1.1%)	—	4(4.2%)
Whitney et al.[20]	279	3(1.1%)	5(1.8%)	6(2.2%)
Javid et al.[21]	65	1(1.5%)	1(1.5%)	1(1.5%)
Anderson et al.[22]	120	0	2(1.7%)	0
VA Clinical Trial[23]	211	4(1.9%)	2(0.9%)	5(2.4%)

symptomatic unilateral carotid stenosis treated by endarterectomy, in many instances with asymptomatic contralateral stenosis noted arteriographically; or the presence of significant stenosis in a patient scheduled for another major operative procedure.

The most common clinical situation is the patient referred with a cervical bruit who either is asymptomatic or has occasional intermittent episodes of nonspecific global symptoms such as light-headedness, dizziness, or perhaps nonspecific visual irregularities. These patients should be referred for noninvasive carotid testing; if the results of testing are positive (area-reducing stenoses of 75% or greater are noted), they should be considered candidates for arteriography and possible endarterectomy. The incidence of these findings is difficult to define for the asymptomatic population, however. Hennerici and colleagues[24] screened more than 2,000 neurologically asymptomatic patients using direct continuous-wave Doppler techniques. Significant extracranial disease was identified in 32.8% of the patients with peripheral vascular disease, in 6.8% of the patients with coronary artery disease, and in 5.9% of the patients with significant risk factors. Moore and associates[25] also reported the results of a survey evaluating the prevalence of carotid artery stenosis in an unselected asymptomatic population older than 50 years of age. Carotid occlusive disease was identified in about 10% of the group. In addition, ste-

TABLE 3.

Incidence of Late Cerebral Events Associated With Asymptomatic Contralateral Stenosis of 50% to 75%*

Authors	Follow-up (yr)	Number of Arteries	Number of Transient Ischemic Attacks (%)	Number of Cerebrovascular Accidents (%)
Podore et al.[26]	5	22	3(14)	2(9)
Humphries et al.[4]	0–13	182†	29(16)	1(0.5)
Durward et al.[27]	4	31	4(13)	0
Levin et al.[5]	0–20	147‡	9(6)	0
Johnson et al.[28]	1–4	22§	2(9)	0
Total		404	47(12)	3(0.7)

*From Long JB, Lynch TG, Hobson RW: Asymptomatic carotid stenosis, in Wilson SE, Veith FJ, Hobson RW, et al (eds): *Vascular Surgery: Principles and Practice.* New York, McGraw-Hill, 1987, pp 581–591.

†Of the arteries, 111 were contralateral to a symptomatic stenosis, 66% had a stenosis measuring between 50% and 70%, 19% had a stenosis between 71% and 90%, and 15% had a stenosis exceeding 90%.

‡Of the arteries, 85% had a stenosis measuring between 50% and 90%, 15% had a stenosis between 91% and 99%, and 8% had nonstenotic ulcerative disease. Five patients had prophylactic repair of the asymptomatic artery before repair of the symptomatic side, and 5 had prophylactic endarterectomy before coronary bypass.

§This series includes arteries with stenoses of 51% to 99%. Both of the transient ischemic attacks were associated with 60% stenoses.

noses of increasing significance were noted with each passing decade of life.

The second clinically important group of patients has asymptomatic carotid stenosis contralateral to a symptomatic lesion that has caused a lateralizing neurologic event. Prior retrospective series have addressed the problem of asymptomatic contralateral stenosis, and data from these series are presented in Table 3. Podore[26] reported data from 67 patients whose arteriograms demonstrated contralateral stenosis, with 42% of the stenoses exceeding 50%. These authors observed an increased incidence of stroke during the clinical follow-up period and concluded that carotid endarterectomy was indicated at centers with a combined perioperative stroke and death rate of less than 3%. Other authors[24, 25, 28] have reported a surprisingly low incidence of stroke in patients with contralateral high-grade asymptomatic stenosis. The results among these patients as reported in a recently published, prospectively randomized clinical trial,[6] however, demonstrated no differences in rates of neurologic events for these two groups. Of additional significance is the fact that these authors[24, 25, 28] included only a few patients with stenoses exceeding 75%, and that some surgeons nonrandomly selected patients with stenoses greater than 75% for endarterectomy. Because clinical data suggest that increased morbidity is associated with increasingly severe stenosis, this selection process may have underestimated the incidence of stroke. Therefore, it appears that stenotic lesions of less than 75% that are opposite symptomatic lesions can be followed clinically. Lesions of greater than 75%, however, must be considered for prophylactic endarterectomy.

CLINICAL TRIALS

Surgical treatment of these two important groups of patients has been influenced by recently published results from prospective, randomized trials.[6, 29] The CASANOVA trial results[29] must be considered inconclusive, as patients with severe stenoses (>90%) were referred for operation and were not included in the randomization protocol. Although no significant reduction occurred in rates of stroke or of stroke and death, additional features of the protocol coupled with exclusion of the patient population at highest risk may have resulted in these indecisive results.

Recent publication of a second prospective, randomized trial conducted within the Veterans Administration,[6] however, has provided additional insight into the treatment of these patients. This multicenter clinical trial was conducted at 11 Department of Veterans Affairs Medical Centers to define the efficacy of carotid endarterectomy on the combined incidence of neurologic outcome events, including TIA, transient monocular blindness, and stroke. Data on 444 adult male patients with asymptomatic carotid stenosis, shown arteriographically to reduce the diameter of the lumen by 50% or more (in the presence of positive results of a Gee-OPG or duplex scan showing 75% area reduction), were examined. Patients were randomized to optimal medical treatment, including aspirin therapy and carotid endarterectomy (n=211) vs. optimal medical treatment alone, including antiplatelet therapy (n=233). All patients were observed independently by a vascular surgeon and a neurologist at each par-

TABLE 4.
Patient Characteristics at Study Entry*†

Patient Characteristics	Surgical Group	Medical Group
Number of patients	211	233
Mean age (SD)	64.1 (6.8)	64.7 (6.7)
Race (%)		
White	88	86
African-American	6	8
Hispanic	1	3
Native American	2	3
Asian-American	2	0
Previous contralateral symptoms (%)	32	33
Daily smoker (%)	52	49
Previous smoker (%)	43	42
History of (%):		
Diabetes	30	27
Myocardial infarct	28	25
Angina pectoris	30	25
Congestive heart failure	5	7
Hypertension	63	64
Arrhythmia	17	14
Peripheral vascular disease	61	59

*From Hobson RW, Weiss DG, Fields WS, et al: N Engl J Med 1993;
328:221–227. Used by permission.
†No significant differences were noted between treatment groups.

ticipating center during a mean follow-up period of 47.9 months. The mean age of the clinical population was 64.5 years and the clinical characteristics of randomized patients at entry are summarized in Table 4. Thirty-two percent of the trial's patients had a history of ischemic events caused by contralateral stenoses, and 80% of these events were reported as TIAs. Two thirds of the sample involved patients with bilateral asymptomatic cerebral hemispheres. Medical exclusionary criteria included previous cerebral infarction, prior endarterectomy with restenosis, previous extracranial-to-intracranial bypass, high surgical risk as a result of associated medical illness, chronic anticoagulant therapy, aspirin intolerance or chronic higher-dose aspirin therapy, life expectancy less than 5 years, surgically inaccessible lesions, noncompliance, or refusal to participate in the protocol.

All patients received initial doses of aspirin at 650 mg twice daily that were reduced to 325 mg daily for those with aspirin intolerance[30, 31] during the subsequent clinical follow-up period. Patients randomized to

TABLE 5.

Combined Neurologic End Points of Transient Ischemic Attack, Transient Monocular Blindness, and Stroke (Nonfatal and Fatal) for Ipsilateral and Contralateral Events*

Neurologic End Point	Surgical Group (n = 211)		Medical Group (n = 233)	
	Number	Percent	Number	Percent
Transient ischemic attack	9	4.3	17	7.3
Transient monocular blindness	1	0.5	12	5.2
Stroke	17	8.1	28	12.0
Total†	27	12.9	57	24.5

*From Hobson RW, Weiss DG, Fields WS, et al: *N Engl J Med* 1993; 328:221–227. Used by permission.
†$P < .002$; relative risk, 0.51; 95% confidence interval: 0.32, 0.81.

carotid endarterectomy underwent operation within 10 days of randomization. Patients who experienced clinically defined neurologic outcome events were evaluated independently by the vascular surgeon and neurologist at each center, and their conclusions were submitted for blinded review and adjudication to the Endpoints Committee. The study initiated enrollment of patients on April 1, 1983, and patient acquisition was completed in October 1987; clinical follow-up ended on March 31, 1991. Mean follow-up as measured from time of entry to first neurologic event, death, or loss to follow-up was 47.9 months.

Morbidity and mortality data for carotid endarterectomy have been published previously.[23] The 30-day operative mortality rate among patients in this study was 1.9% (4 of 211 patients), with three deaths result-

TABLE 6.

Combined Neurologic End Points of Transient Ischemic Attack, Transient Monocular Blindness, and Stroke (Nonfatal and Fatal) for Ipsilateral Events Only*

Neurologic End Point	Surgical Group (n = 211)		Medical Group (n = 233)	
	Number	Percent	Number	Percent
Transient ischemic attack	6	2.8	15	6.4
Transient monocular blindness	1	0.5	11	4.7
Stroke†	10	4.7	22	9.4
Total‡	17	8.0	48	20.6

*From Hobson RW, Weiss DG, Fields WS, et al: *N Engl J Med* 1993; 328:221–227. Used by permission.
†$P = .056$.
‡$P < .001$; relative risk, 0.38; 95% confidence interval: 0.22, 0.67.

ing from myocardial infarction and one from myocardial infarction followed by stroke. Five postoperative strokes (nonfatal) occurred, for an incidence of 2.4% (5 of 211 patients). Three nonfatal strokes (0.4%, 3 of 714 patients) occurred as a result of arteriography; one was associated with significant hemiparesis (0.15%) and two were associated with minimal neurologic deficits. The 30-day rate of permanent stroke and death after randomization was 4.7% for the surgical group, assigning all complications of arteriography for this trial to the surgical group. In contrast, during the first 30 days after assignment of patients to the medical group, one death as a result of suicide (0.4%) and two neurologic events (0.9%) occurred (one permanent stroke and one transient ischemic event).

The results for all neurologic events, both contralateral and ipsilateral, are summarized in Table 5. Eighty-four events were observed, 27 (12.9%) in the surgical group and 57 (24.5%) in the medical group, which represented an absolute risk reduction of 11.6% ($P < .002$) and a relative (surgical-to-medical) risk of 0.51 (95% confidence interval: 0.32, 0.81). Results for ipsilateral events only are presented in Table 6. There were 65 ipsilateral events, 17 (8.0%) in the surgical group and 48 (20.6%) in the

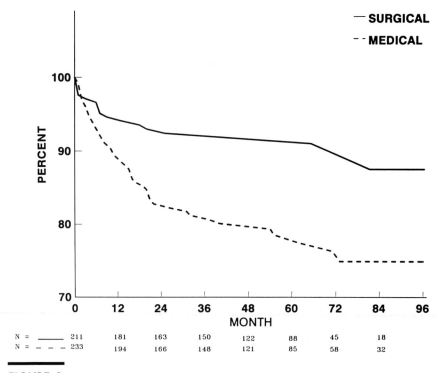

FIGURE 2.

Event-free rates for first ipsilateral stroke and transient ischemic attack, including transient monocular blindness. Kaplan-Meier curves of an analysis of the time until the occurrence of the first event for surgical and medical groups. The numbers (N) of patients remaining event-free and on study at the beginning of each 12-month period are provided under the graph. Treatment group comparisons by the log-rank test demonstrated significant differences in favor of the surgical group ($P < .001$). The relative risk (surgical vs. medical) was 0.38 (95% confidence interval: 0.22, 0.67). (From Hobson RW, Weiss DG, Fields WS, et al: *N Engl J Med* 1993; 328:221–227. Used by permission.)

medical group. The absolute risk reduction was 12.6% ($P < .001$), for a relative risk of 0.38 (95% confidence interval: 0.22, 0.67). Analysis of ipsilateral neurologic events in the medical group revealed 24 events (19.2%; 12 strokes, 7 TIAs, 5 episodes of transient monocular blindness) among patients with stenoses of 50% to 75%, and 24 events (22.4%; 10 strokes, 8 TIAs, 6 episodes of transient monocular blindness) among those with stenoses of 76% to 99%, which did not represent a significant difference.

The temporal distribution of neurologic outcome events over the duration of follow-up was determined by the construction of Kaplan-Meier survival curves, in which survival was defined as the time until the first neurologic event occurred. Data for ipsilateral events are summarized in Figure 2. The numbers of patients remaining event free and on study at the beginning of each 12-month interval are provided under the graph. Treatment group comparisons by the log-rank test demonstrated significant differences in favor of the surgical group ($P < .001$).

The incidence of stroke and death for this high-risk group of patients is presented in Table 7. No significant differences were observed between treatment groups.

The results of this clinical trial[16] indicate that carotid endarterectomy combined with optimal medical treatment can reduce the incidence of ipsilateral neurologic outcome events in high-risk male patients with arteriographically confirmed asymptomatic carotid stenosis. In addition, the incidence of ipsilateral stroke alone was reduced significantly ($P = .056$) in the surgically treated group. When the four perioperative deaths (1.9%) were added to this analysis, however, the 30-day perioperative stroke and death rates were not significantly different between groups. Emphasizing the importance of maintaining low perioperative complication rates among surgically treated patients,[32] our current preoperative work-up includes a rigorous evaluation of the coronary circulation using

TABLE 7.
Stroke, Stroke Death, and All Other Deaths*†

Cause of Death	Surgical Group (n = 211)		Medical Group (n = 233)	
	Number	Percent	Number	Percent
Nonfatal stroke	17	8.0	25	10.7
Stroke death	1	0.5	4	1.7
Myocardial infarction/cardiac/sudden‡	44	20.9	47	20.2
Other medical	19	9.0	17	7.3
Unknown	6	2.8	10	4.3
Total†	87	41.2	103	44.2

*From Hobson RW, Weiss DG, Fields WS, et al: *N Engl J Med* 1993; 328:221–227. Used by permission.
†No significant difference was noted (relative risk, 0.92; 95% confidence interval: 0.69, 1.22).
‡Includes 4 perioperative deaths.

thallium scans as indicated. Carotid endarterectomy is recommended for patients with high-grade asymptomatic stenosis who have received surgical clearance in regard to coronary artery disease and are expected to live 5 years or more. Although this trial was unable to demonstrate the influence of carotid endarterectomy on the combined incidence of stroke and death, a modest effect could not be excluded because of the sample size. Data from the Asymptomatic Carotid Atherosclerosis Study,[33] however, which has an anticipated sample size of 1,500 patients, may be able to address this important question.

The third clinically important group of patients are those who are identified as having asymptomatic carotid stenoses during preoperative evaluation for major general surgical or cardiovascular operative procedures. Intraoperative hypotension combined with carotid stenosis may predispose a patient to carotid arterial occlusion and has been suggested as a mechanism for the development of stroke. Nevertheless, the overall risk of perioperative stroke is only 0.3% to 0.5% in patients undergoing general surgery, 1% to 2% in those undergoing vascular surgical procedures, and 2% to 5% in those undergoing coronary bypass grafting.[34] Although there is no well-documented relationship between the presence of a carotid bruit and the subsequent incidence of perioperative stroke, the perioperative risk of stroke in asymptomatic patients with stenoses of 75% or greater has not been evaluated fully yet. Barnes and coworkers[35] used spectral analysis and cerebrovascular Doppler examinations to evaluate 449 patients undergoing carotid or peripheral vascular operations. Fourteen percent of the patients had carotid stenoses that exceeded 50% of the arterial diameter; however, the range and distribution of these stenoses were not detailed. Nevertheless, no correlation between the presence of carotid stenosis and the incidence of perioperative stroke was reported. The incidence of postoperative death from myocardial infarction, though, was increased significantly in this group of patients. Brener and associates[36] used noninvasive techniques to study 2,026 patients before they underwent coronary bypass. Fifty patients (2.5%) were identified as having hemodynamically significant stenoses. Although this is significantly less than the 12.3% reported by Barnes[35] or the 11.8% reported by Turnipseed and colleagues,[37] a 15% incidence of perioperative neurologic deficit was noted in patients with significant carotid occlusive disease compared with a 2% incidence in patients without significant stenoses. Nevertheless, Brener recommended against prophylactic endarterectomy in this population because of the high incidence of perioperative complications associated with the combined endarterectomy and aortocoronary bypass procedure. The decision to perform a prophylactic endarterectomy before a major operative procedure must be based on the magnitude of the stenotic disease and the associated risk of endarterectomy. Although the overall incidence of stroke associated with aortic reconstruction or coronary bypass procedures is low, operative intervention may be appropriate in patients with stenosis of 75% or greater, or in those with significant bilateral disease. We recommend combined procedures only for asymptomatic patients with bilateral area stenoses of 75% or greater, or with a comparable unilateral stenosis coupled with a contralateral asymptomatic occlusion. Whether concomitant carotid endarterectomy reduces the incidence of perioperative stroke in these patients remains controversial. Subsequent or staged endarterectomy once the patient has recovered from the cardiac surgical procedure may be indicated, however, as a part of a program of long-term stroke prevention. Furthermore, the Asymptomatic Carotid Atherosclerosis Study group[33] is interested in examining this question in a prospective, randomized fashion. Until this can be accomplished, no precise conclusion regarding this group of patients is possible.

CURRENT RECOMMENDATIONS

Retrospective and prospective clinical analyses have demonstrated that carotid endarterectomy combined with optimal medical treatment can reduce the incidence of ipsilateral neurologic outcome events in high-risk patients with arteriographically confirmed asymptomatic carotid stenosis. Despite the enhanced risk of TIA and stroke for this population of patients, however, most will die as a result of coronary atherosclerosis. Consequently, care must be exercised in the selection of patients for operation. Acceptably low perioperative complication rates (see Table 2) should be confirmed by clinical audit at each institution before a program of operative intervention is instituted. Although the Veterans Administration trial demonstrated a trend toward reduction in stroke alone (see Table 6), the more definitive analysis of stroke plus death must await the publication of results from the National Institutes of Health–sponsored Asymptomatic Carotid Atherosclerosis Study, with its anticipated larger sample size of 1,500 patients. For participants in this trial, its program of clinical follow-up is recommended. For those patients who are unwilling or unable to participate, however, carotid endarterectomy offers important advantages for selected individuals whose surgeons have demonstrated low complication rates.

REFERENCES

1. NASCET Collaborators: Beneficial effect of carotid endarterectomy in symptomatic patients with high-grade carotid stenosis. N Engl J Med 1991; 325:445–453.
2. European Carotid Surgery Trialists' (ECST) Collaborative Group: MRC European Carotid Surgery interim results for symptomatic patients with severe (70–99%) or mild (0–29%) carotid stenosis. Lancet 1991; 337:1235–1243.
3. Mayberg MR, Wilson SE, Yatsu F, et al: Carotid endarterectomy and prevention of cerebral ischemia in symptomatic carotid stenosis. JAMA 1991; 266:3289–3294.
4. Humphries AW, Young JR, Santilli PA, et al: Unoperated asymptomatic significant internal carotid artery stenosis: A review of 182 instances. Surgery 1976; 80:695–698.
5. Levin SM, Sondheimer FK, Levin JM: The contralateral diseased but asymptomatic carotid artery: To operate or not? An update. Am J Surg 1980; 140: 203–205.
6. Hobson RW, Weiss DG, and the Veterans Affairs Cooperative Study Group: Efficacy of carotid endarterectomy for asymptomatic carotid stenosis. N Engl J Med 1993; 328:221–227.

7. Norris JW: Outcome in patients with asymptomatic carotid stenosis, in *Consensus Conference on the Management of Asymptomatic Carotid Stenosis*, in press.

8. Toole J, Hobson RW, Howard VJ, et al: Nearing the finish line? The Asymptomatic Carotid Atherosclerosis Study (editorial). *Stroke* 1992; 23:1054–1055.

9. Wolf PA, Kannel WB, Sorlie P, et al: Asymptomatic carotid bruit and the risk of stroke. *JAMA* 1981; 245:1442–1445.

10. Heyman W, Wilkinson WE, Heyden S, et al: Risk of stroke in asymptomatic persons with cervical arterial bruits. A population study in Evans County, Georgia. *N Engl J Med* 1980; 302:838–841.

11. Norris JW, Zhu CZ, Bornstein NM, et al: Vascular risks of asymptomatic carotid stenosis. *Stroke* 1991; 22:485.

12. Gee W, Mehigan JT, Wylie EJ: Measurement of collateral cerebral hemispheric blood pressure by ocular pneumoplethysmography. *Am J Surg* 1975; 130:121–127.

13. Blackshear WM Jr, Phillips DJ, Thiele BL, et al: Detection of carotid occlusive disease by ultrasonic imaging and pulsed Doppler spectrum analysis. *Surgery* 1979; 86:698–706.

14. Hobson RW, Song IS, George AM, et al: Results of arteriography for asymptomatic carotid stenosis. *Stroke* 1989; 20:135.

15. Toole JF: The Willis Lecture: Transient ischemic attacks, scientific method, and new realities. *Stroke* 1991; 22:99–104.

16. Norris JW, Zhu CZ: Silent stroke and carotid stenosis. *Stroke* 1992; 23:483.

17. Thompson JE, Patman RD, Talkington CM: Asymptomatic carotid bruit: Long-term outcome in patients having endarterectomy compared with unoperated controls. *Ann Surg* 1978; 188:308–316.

18. Moore WS, Boren C, Malone JM, et al: Asymptomatic carotid stenosis: Immediate and long-term results after prophylactic endarterectomy. *Am J Surg* 1979; 138:228–233.

19. Hertzer NR, Beven EG, Greenstreet RL, et al: Internal carotid back pressures, intraoperative shunting, ulcerated atheromata, and the incidence of stroke during carotid endarterectomy. *Surgery* 1978; 83:306–312.

20. Whitney DG, Kahn EM, Estes JW, et al: Carotid artery surgery without a temporary indwelling shunt. *Arch Surg* 1980; 115:1393–1399.

21. Javid H, Ostermiller WE, Hengesh JW, et al: Carotid endarterectomy for asymptomatic patients. *Arch Surg* 1971; 102:389–391.

22. Anderson RJ, Hobson RW, Padberg FT, et al: Carotid endarterectomy for asymptomatic carotid stenosis: A ten year experience with 120 procedures in a fellowship training program. *Ann Vasc Surg* 1991; 5:111–115.

23. Towne JB, Weiss DG, Hobson RW: First phase report of Veterans Administration asymptomatic carotid stenosis study—operative morbidity and mortality. *J Vasc Surg* 1990; 11:252–259.

24. Hennerici M, Aulich A, Sandman W, et al: Incidence of asymptomatic extracranial disease. *Stroke* 1981; 12:750–758.

25. Moore DJ, Sheehan MP, Kolm P, et al: Are strokes predictable with noninvasive methods: A five year follow-up of 303 unoperated patients. *J Vasc Surg* 1985; 2:654–660.

26. Podore PC, DeWeese JA, May AG, et al: Asymptomatic contralateral carotid endarterectomy. *Surgery* 1980; 88:748–752.

27. Durward QJ, Ferguson GG, Barr HWK: The natural history of asymptomatic carotid bifurcation plaques. *Stroke* 1982; 13:459–464.

28. Johnson N, Burnham SJ, Flanigan DP, et al: Carotid endarterectomy: A follow-up study of the contralateral nonoperated carotid artery. *Ann Surg* 1978; 188:748–752.

29. CASANOVA Study Group: Carotid surgery versus medical therapy in asymptomatic carotid stenosis. *Stroke* 1991; 22:1229–1235.
30. Krupski WC, Weiss DG, and the VA Cooperative Asymptomatic Carotid Artery Stenosis Study Group: Adverse effects of aspirin in the treatment of asymptomatic carotid artery stenosis. *J Vasc Surg* 1992; 16:588–600.
31. Hobson RW, Krupski WC, Weiss DG, and the VA Cooperative Asymptomatic Carotid Artery Stenosis Study Group: Influence of aspirin in the management of asymptomatic carotid stenosis. *J Vasc Surg*, 1993; 17:257–265.
32. Hobson RW, Towne J: Carotid endarterectomy for asymptomatic carotid stenosis (editorial). *Stroke* 1989; 20:575–576.
33. The Asymptomatic Carotid Atherosclerosis Study Group: Study design for randomized prospective trial of carotid endarterectomy for asymptomatic atherosclerosis. *Stroke* 1989; 20:844–849.
34. Long JB, Lynch TG, Hobson RW: Asymptomatic carotid stenosis, in Wilson SE, Veith FJ, Hobson RW, et al (eds): *Vascular Surgery: Principles and Practices.* New York, McGraw-Hill, 1987, pp 581–591.
35. Barnes RW, Liebman PR, Marszalek PB, et al: The natural history of asymptomatic carotid disease in patients undergoing cardiovascular surgery. *Surgery* 1981; 90:1075–1083.
36. Brener BJ, Brief DK, Alpert J, et al: A four-year experience with preoperative noninvasive carotid evaluation of two thousand twenty-six patients undergoing cardiac surgery. *J Vasc Surg* 1984; 1:326–338.
37. Turnipseed WD, Berkoff HA, Belzer FO: Postoperative stroke in cardiac and peripheral vascular disease. *Ann Surg* 1980; 192:365–368.
38. Lynch TG, Hobson RW: Noninvasive cerebrovascular diagnostic techniques, in Wilson SE, Veith FJ, Hobson RW, et al (eds): *Vascular Surgery: Principles and Practice.* New York, McGraw-Hill, 1987, pp 105–134.

Diagnostic Evaluation of Carotid Artery Disease

R. EUGENE ZIERLER, M.D.

T he first description of cerebral arteriography in a living patient was reported by Moniz in 1927, and arteriography remained the only objective diagnostic method for classifying the severity of carotid artery disease until the introduction of noninvasive testing almost 50 years later.[1, 2] Although arteriography provides accurate anatomic information, its high cost and invasive nature make it unsuitable for use as a screening test or for performing serial follow-up examinations. Furthermore, arteriography does not indicate the physiologic consequences of arterial lesions. During the past 2 decades, the risks and limitations of arteriography have stimulated the development of noninvasive methods for the evaluation of carotid artery disease. Since these tests are characterized by minimal risk, absence of patient discomfort, and relatively low cost, they can be used to document both the extent of disease at one point in time and the subsequent changes that occur. In addition, other less invasive radiologic imaging methods have been developed since the advent of arteriography that also have applications in the diagnosis and management of carotid artery disease. This article will review the current status of the noninvasive and radiologic methods for the diagnostic evaluation of carotid artery disease.

NONINVASIVE DIAGNOSTIC METHODS

The noninvasive tests for carotid artery disease can be considered as either indirect or direct (Table 1). The first tests to be applied in the clinical setting were indirect tests such as the periorbital Doppler examination.[2] Although the indirect tests still may be of value in selected patients, the direct approach of duplex scanning clearly is the current method of choice for routine clinical applications.

INDIRECT TESTS

The indirect tests rely on changes in pressure or flow in the distal branches of the internal and external carotid arteries to indicate the presence of lesions at the carotid bifurcation.[3] However, because pressure and flow in the carotid system do not fall until the diameter of the lumen is reduced by 50% or more, the indirect tests can detect only severe stenoses and occlusions. Consequently, these tests cannot distinguish between normal and minimally diseased arteries or differentiate occlusion from

Advances in Vascular Surgery, vol. 1.
©1993, Mosby–Year Book, Inc.

TABLE 1.

Noninvasive Tests for Carotid Artery Disease

I. Indirect tests
   A. Periorbital Doppler examination
   B. Oculoplethysmography
      1. Fluid-filled
      2. Air-filled (OPG-GEE)
II. Direct tests
   A. Ultrasonic arteriography
   B. B-mode imaging
   C. Duplex scanning
      1. B-mode imaging
      2. Pulsed Doppler flow detection
      3. Spectral waveform analysis
      4. Color-flow imaging
   D. Transcranial Doppler

high-grade stenosis. Since the test results typically are reported as either positive or negative, these methods are of limited value in classifying the relative severity of carotid lesions and in monitoring disease progression.

Periorbital Doppler Examination

The ophthalmic artery is the first intracranial branch of the internal carotid, and the periorbital Doppler examination demonstrates the direction of flow in the branches of the ophthalmic artery that supply the periorbital area of the face. Thus, proximal occlusive disease in the carotid system can be evaluated by detecting changes in blood flow patterns around the eye. Blood flow in the periorbital arteries normally moves from the inside to the outside of the orbit. In the presence of severe stenosis or occlusion of the internal carotid artery, the periorbital branches of the external carotid and the ophthalmic artery can serve as an important collateral route to the ipsilateral cerebral hemisphere. When this occurs, reversal of flow is found in the periorbital arteries, and sources of collateral flow can be identified by a series of compression maneuvers. The principal advantage of the periorbital Doppler test is that it requires inexpensive equipment and is relatively simple to perform. An abnormal test is a good indicator of a hemodynamically significant carotid lesion; however, false-negative results are common and tend to be associated with common or external carotid stenoses and efficient collateral pathways.[4] Thus, this test is most reliable when it is abnormal.

Oculoplethysmography

In the presence of a carotid lesion that reduces distal pressure or flow, the collateral pathways may result in a delay of the ocular pulse or a reduction in the ocular perfusion pressure. Kartchner and McRae described an indirect test based on detecting the difference in pulse arrival times between the two eyes.[5] The ocular pulsations were sensed through saline-filled tubes connected to small plastic cups applied to the corneas, and external carotid pulsations were detected by a photoplethysmograph transducer clipped to each ear. Pulse waveforms from the eyes and ears were compared electronically and any delay or distortion was noted. Because of the extremely variable and inconsistent results reported with fluid-filled oculoplethysmograph, this method generally is considered to be unsuitable for routine diagnosis.

The most widely used oculoplethysmographic method is the air-filled system developed by Gee.[6] This instrument measures ophthalmic artery pressure through small suction cups placed on the sclera lateral to the corneas. Ocular pulsations are obliterated temporarily by applying a negative pressure of 300 to 500 mm Hg to the cups, and the pressure in the system is decreased gradually until the pulsations reappear. Criteria for interpretation are based on the difference between the pressures in the two eyes and the relationship between ophthalmic and brachial artery pressures. This approach has a relatively high accuracy for detecting carotid lesions of more than about 65% diameter reduction. In addition, the false-negative rate generally is lower than that seen with the periorbital Doppler examination.

DIRECT TESTS

With the direct tests, diagnostic information is obtained from the carotid artery segment where the lesions of interest are located. Strictly speaking, the direct tests include such methods as carotid phonoangiography, quantitative phonoangiography, the continuous-wave Doppler scan, and ultrasonic arteriography.[3] However, the techniques that combine B-mode imaging and pulsed Doppler ultrasound have emerged as the most accurate and reliable for classification of carotid artery disease.

B-Mode Imaging

B-mode imaging has been used to evaluate the histologic and surface features of carotid lesions with varying degrees of success.[7-9] Although the sonographic characteristics of a plaque may correlate qualitatively with its histologic composition, the clinical value of this information has not been established clearly. In general, lipid is the least echogenic component of atherosclerotic plaque. As the collagen content of a plaque increases relative to its lipid content, the echogenicity also increases. Fibrous plaque usually is homogeneous, but focal deposits of thrombus or lipid can produce a more heterogeneous appearance. Calcification, which typically occurs at sites of hemorrhage or necrosis, is extremely echogenic and results in bright echoes with acoustic shadows (Fig 1). The sonographic characteristic of plaque that appears to be most related to clinical outcome is heterogeneity.[10] This feature has been attributed to intraplaque hemorrhage, which has been found more frequently in symptomatic than asymptomatic patients.[11]

Since ulcerated plaque commonly is regarded as a source of cerebral emboli, there has been considerable interest in the sonographic evaluation of plaque surface characteristics. Although some favorable results have been reported, the reliability of B-mode imaging for the detection of ulcerated atherosclerotic plaque generally has been poor.[9, 11, 12] Experience with B-mode imaging alone for the classification of carotid artery disease has shown that the image is most accurate for lesions of minimal to moderate severity and least accurate for high-grade stenoses or occlu-

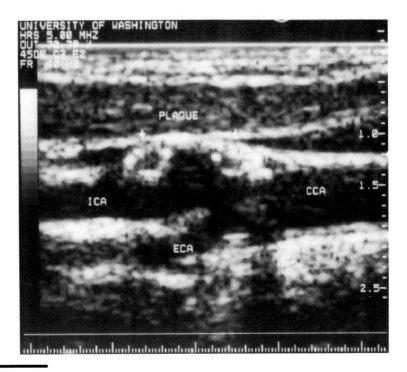

FIGURE 1.

B-mode image of a carotid bifurcation plaque. A calcified plaque is present along the near wall of the carotid bulb, indicated by the *arrows*, with acoustic shadowing in the distal common carotid artery *(CCA)*. *ICA* = internal carotid artery; *ECA* = external carotid artery.

sions.[8] However, it often is difficult to determine the size of the arterial lumen using a B-mode image because the acoustic properties of noncalcified plaque, thrombus, and flowing blood are similar. In addition, acoustic shadows from calcified plaques may prevent complete visualization of the arterial wall. These limitations largely are overcome by duplex scanning.

Duplex Scanning

The concept of combining B-mode imaging and pulsed Doppler flow detection in a single instrument was developed when it became apparent that B-mode imaging alone was not a satisfactory method for determining the severity of arterial disease. This method, which became known as duplex scanning, made it possible to obtain anatomic and physiologic information directly from selected sites within the vascular system. The duplex approach is based on the concept that arterial lesions produce disturbances in blood flow patterns that can be characterized by analysis of Doppler flow signals. In conventional duplex scanning, vessels are visualized on the B-mode image and a single pulsed Doppler sample volume is placed within the arterial lumen at a site of interest. The local flow pattern then is assessed by spectral waveform analysis. Although the B-mode image may be useful for identifying anatomic variants and arterial wall thickening or calcification, the classification of disease severity

TABLE 2.

Criteria for Classification of Internal Carotid Artery Disease by Duplex Scanning With Spectral Waveform Analysis of Pulsed Doppler Signals

Arteriographic Lesion	Spectral Criteria*
A. 0% diameter reduction	Peak systolic frequency less than 4 kHz; no spectral broadening
B. 1% to 15% diameter reduction	Peak systolic frequency less than 4 kHz; spectral broadening in deceleration phase of systole only
C. 16% to 49% diameter reduction	Peak systolic frequency less than 4 kHz; spectral broadening throughout systole
D. 50% to 79% diameter reduction	Peak systolic frequency greater than or equal to 4 kHz; end-diastolic frequency less than 4.5 kHz
D+. 80% to 99% diameter reduction	End-diastolic frequency greater than or equal to 4.5 kHz
E. Occlusion (100% diameter reduction)	No internal carotid flow signal; flow to zero in common carotid artery

*Criteria are based on a pulsed Doppler with a 5-MHz transmitting frequency, a sample volume that is small relative to the internal carotid artery, and a 60-degree beam-to-vessel angle of insonation. Approximate angle-adjusted velocity equivalents are 4 kHz = 125 cm/sec and 4.5 kHz = 140 cm/sec.

is based primarily on interpretation of pulsed Doppler spectral waveforms.

The spectral waveform features used to classify carotid lesions include spectral broadening, which represents turbulent flow, and increased peak systolic frequency, which results from the high-velocity jet within a stenosis. Spectral waveform criteria for classification of internal carotid artery stenoses have been validated by a series of comparisons with contrast arteriograms.[13–15] A set of currently used criteria is given in Table 2 and illustrated in Figure 2. These criteria distinguish between normal and diseased internal carotid arteries with a specificity of 84% and a sensitivity of 99%. The accuracy for detecting 50% to 99% diameter stenosis or occlusion is 93%.

Some variability is unavoidable in the performance and interpretation of physiologic or anatomic tests. In carotid duplex scanning, the greatest variability has been noted for the normal to moderate stenosis categories, which are designated as A, B, and C lesions in Table 2. Agreement is much better for classification of lesions that are greater than 50% diameter reducing.[16] Similarly, carotid arteriography is subject to the most variability when the arteries are normal or minimally diseased.[17] In general, the agreement between duplex scanning and arteriography is equivalent to the agreement between two radiologists interpreting the same arteriograms.

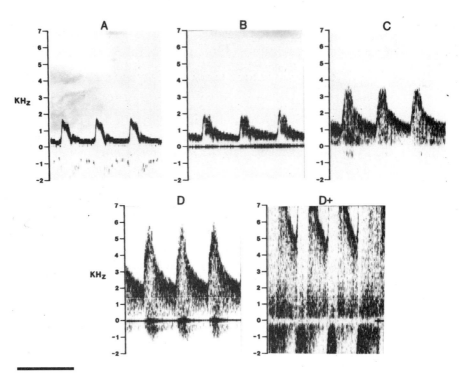

FIGURE 2.

Examples of internal carotid spectral waveforms classified according to the criteria given in Table 2. **A,** normal; **B,** 1% to 15% diameter reduction; **C,** 16% to 49% diameter reduction; **D,** 50% to 79% diameter reduction; **D +,** 80% to 99% diameter reduction. (From Zierler RE, Strandness DE Jr: Noninvasive dynamic and real-time assessment of extracranial cerebrovasculature, in Wood JH (ed): *Cerebral Blood Flow: Physiologic and Clinical Aspects.* New York, McGraw-Hill, 1987, p 317. Used by permission.)

Color-Flow Imaging

Color-flow imaging is an alternative to spectral waveform analysis for displaying the Doppler information obtained by duplex scanning. Within certain technical limitations, the color-flow image permits visualization of moving blood in the plane of the B-mode image (Fig 3). Whereas spectral analysis displays the entire frequency and amplitude content of the signal at a selected site, color-flow imaging provides a single estimate of the Doppler shift frequency or flow velocity for each site within the B-mode image. Thus, spectral waveforms actually give considerably more information on flow at each individual site than does color-flow imaging. The principal advantage of the color-flow display is that it presents flow information on the entire image, even though the amount of information on each site is reduced. Color-flow imaging can be extremely helpful for identifying vessels, particularly when they are small, deeply located, or anatomically complex (Fig 4).[18] Changes in the color-flow image also may show areas of flow separation that are characteristic of the normal carotid bulb or flow disturbances associated with arterial disease. Since the color assignments in the flow image represent mean rather than peak velocities, however, it is difficult to determine disease severity based on the

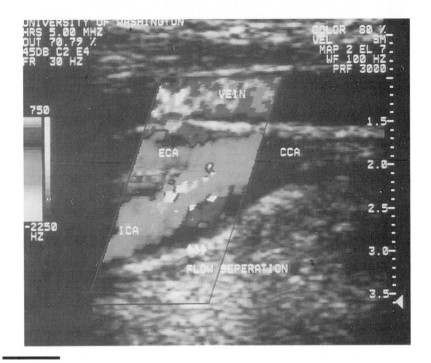

FIGURE 3.

Black and white representation of a color-flow image of a carotid bifurcation showing flow in the distal common (CCA), proximal internal (ICA), and external (ECA) carotid arteries. An area of flow separation, which appears as a dark oval, is present along the outer wall of the carotid bulb.

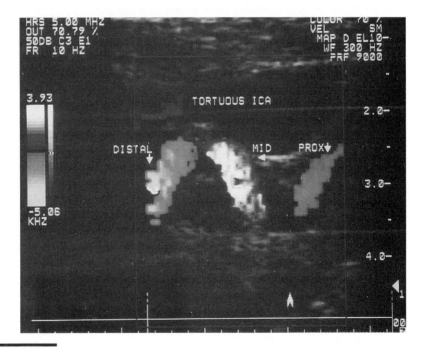

FIGURE 4.

Black and white representation of a color-flow image of a tortuous internal carotid artery (ICA). Color changes result from different angles between the flow stream and the ultrasound scan lines. No color appears when the angle approaches 90 degrees.

color-flow image alone. Therefore, even when color-flow imaging is used, spectral waveforms still are necessary for accurate disease classification.

Transcranial Doppler

Examinations of the extracranial carotid vessels can be performed with ultrasound transmitting frequencies in the range of 3 to 10 MHz, but these frequencies do not penetrate bone sufficiently to reach the intracranial arteries. In 1982, Aaslid reported that flow signals could be acquired from the middle and anterior cerebral arteries with a 2-MHz pulsed Doppler ultrasound beam directed through the temporal bone just above the zygomatic arch.[19] Since that time, the transcranial Doppler examination has developed into a complex technique using not only the temporal window to gain access to the intracranial vessels, but also the orbital window and the foramen magnum.[20] With these additional approaches, the intracranial internal carotid, posterior cerebral, ophthalmic, intracranial vertebral, and basilar arteries can be insonated.

The transcranial Doppler examination relies on the same general principles as the extracranial pulsed Doppler evaluation performed as part of a carotid duplex scan, with diagnostic conclusions based on the changes in flow velocity and direction in the intracranial arteries. Although the transcranial Doppler findings do not permit accurate classification of extracranial carotid disease, there is an inverse correlation between middle cerebral artery flow velocity and the severity of internal carotid artery disease as documented by duplex scanning.[21] Stenoses of the intracranial arteries are indicated by a focal increase in peak velocity followed by a fall in velocity immediately distal to the stenotic segment. Large increases in flow velocity also occur in the vicinity of intracranial arteriovenous malformations; however, these velocity changes are not as focal as those related to stenoses and are present throughout the course of the involved arteries. Potential sources of intracranial collateral flow can be identified by noting the response of various intracranial arteries to common carotid artery compression maneuvers. A fixed transcranial Doppler probe over the temporal window can be used to monitor middle cerebral artery flow during carotid endarterectomy.[21] Middle cerebral artery flow velocity decreases with intraoperative carotid cross-clamping and correlates directly with measured internal carotid stump pressure and electroencephalographic signs of cerebral ischemia. The transcranial Doppler also can be used to document the efficacy of intraoperative shunt function.

Additional applications of transcranial Doppler include the early detection of cerebral vasospasm associated with subarachnoid hemorrhage. Since increased intracranial flow velocities occur prior to neurologic deterioration, this finding allows prompt institution of appropriate therapy. Documentation of flow direction in the vertebral and basilar arteries by transcranial Doppler is helpful in the evaluation of patients with suspected subclavian steal syndrome. The detection of middle cerebral artery emboli by transcranial Doppler has been described recently, suggesting that this technique could be used to guide the management of patients at risk for stroke.[22] Finally, a distinctive high-resistance flow pattern has been noted by transcranial Doppler in cases of brain death. The various clinical applications of transcranial Doppler are summarized in Table 3.

TABLE 3.

Applications of Transcranial Doppler Ultrasonography

Detecting severe stenoses in the major intracranial arteries
Assessing the intracranial collateral circulation in patients with
  extracranial carotid artery disease
Evaluating for cerebral vasospasm, particularly in patients with
  subarachnoid hemorrhage
Detecting arteriovenous malformations
Monitoring intracranial arterial flow during carotid endarterectomy and
  other procedures affecting the cerebral circulation
Evaluating subclavian steal syndrome
Detecting intracranial arterial emboli
Documenting brain death

RADIOLOGIC DIAGNOSTIC METHODS

Since it first was described over 60 years ago, contrast arteriography has
been the standard test for evaluating both the extracranial and intracranial carotid vessels. However, even with the numerous technical improvements that have made arteriography safer, its use still is justified only
when there are compelling clinical indications. With the development of
less invasive radiologic techniques for assessing the cerebral circulation,
the separation between noninvasive and invasive methods has become
less distinct. Although the emphasis of this review has been on the noninvasive approaches, it is worthwhile to comment briefly on the important radiologic techniques.

CONVENTIONAL CONTRAST ARTERIOGRAPHY

There is little doubt that standard contrast arteriography provides the
most accurate and clinically valuable anatomic information on the location and extent of arterial disease. The main disadvantage of conventional
arteriography always has been the risk of complications related to the arterial puncture and contrast injection. Puncture site complications such
as hematoma, false aneurysm, or arterial thrombosis occur in approxi-
mately 5% of cases.[23] The prevalence of neurologic complications following arteriography in patients with cerebrovascular disease also is in the
range of 5%, with less than 1% being permanent. Other rare but significant complications include anaphylactic reactions and contrast-induced
renal failure. Whereas anaphylactic and other allergic reactions to radiographic contrast material are not related to the amount of contrast given,
the risk of renal toxicity does appear to be dose-related. Other factors that
increase the risk of renal dysfunction after arteriography are prior abnormal renal function, abdominal aortic injection site, congestive heart failure, and advanced age.[24]

The risk of puncture site complications can be avoided by using an
intravenous injection of contrast material and digital subtraction tech-

niques to visualize the extracranial carotid system. Although intravenous digital subtraction arteriography can provide useful diagnostic information, the images are uninterpretable in about 10% of studies, and the overall accuracy compared to conventional arteriography is not significantly better than that of carotid duplex scanning.[25, 26] Because of these limitations, this radiologic approach is used seldom.

Although conventional contrast arteriography always has been used to validate the results of noninvasive tests, it should be emphasized that arteriography and noninvasive tests are fundamentally different. Arteriography is strictly an anatomic investigation; duplex scanning and the other noninvasive methods are physiologic tests that detect the hemodynamic effects of arterial disease. Thus, although they tend to be considered as competitive, they actually are complementary in many respects.

COMPUTERIZED CEREBRAL TOMOGRAPHY

The purpose of computerized cerebral tomography in the evaluation of patients with carotid artery disease is to identify intracranial abnormalities that may influence therapeutic decisions. Intracranial lesions include aneurysms, arteriovenous malformations, tumors, and areas of hemorrhage or infarction. The ability of computerized cerebral tomography to detect infarctions is related to the age of the lesions and may be improved by administration of intravenous radiographic contrast. Widespread use of this technique prior to carotid endarterectomy has shown a remarkably high prevalence of infarctions in patients without fixed neurologic deficits. In a review of 359 patients undergoing carotid endarterectomy, preoperative computerized cerebral tomography revealed ipsilateral infarction in 146 (41%), including 76% of those with strokes, 33% with transient ischemic attacks, 23% with nonhemispheric symptoms, and 20% with asymptomatic high-grade carotid stenoses.[27]

MAGNETIC RESONANCE ANGIOGRAPHY

The application of magnetic resonance imaging to the diagnosis of vascular problems is appealing because it would be possible during a single imaging session to evaluate the flow conditions within the vessels of interest, the characteristics of the vessel walls, and the features of surrounding tissues. Magnetic resonance methods are considered noninvasive; however, unlike B-mode ultrasound, they can be used to assess the intracranial and intrathoracic vessels. Although the detailed physical principles of magnetic resonance imaging are beyond the scope of this review, it is appropriate to mention a few technical points. Magnetic resonance images are generated by determining the distribution of hydrogen nuclei or single protons in a volume of tissue. This is accomplished by analyzing the response of the hydrogen nuclei to the presence of a magnetic field and the introduction of energy in the form of radiofrequency waves. The density of hydrogen nuclei within various tissues depends primarily on their water and fat content, so magnetic resonance images tend to reflect the distribution of water and fat.

When a volume of tissue is placed in a strong magnetic field, the magnetic moments of the hydrogen nuclei become aligned with the field. If the tissue then is subjected to a radiofrequency pulse, the hydrogen nuclei absorb energy and are tipped out of alignment with the magnetic field. This additional energy is lost over time as the tipped nuclei realign with the magnetic field and return to their original energy state. A signal is emitted from the tissue as this process takes place, which is detected by an array of sensors and used to construct the magnetic resonance images. The specific features of the images are dependent on the choice of imaging parameters, including the radiofrequency pulse strength, the time interval between radiofrequency pulses, and the interval between radiofrequency transmission and signal detection.[28]

Magnetic resonance angiography is based on the application of magnetic resonance techniques to the detection of flowing blood. In the most commonly used approach, a thin slice of tissue is exposed to a rapid sequence of radiofrequency pulses. Since the stationary components of the tissue never have time to realign with the magnetic field, their signal strength is relatively low. However, blood flowing through the tissue is replenished constantly from outside the plane of excitation and produces a much stronger signal. This process is called "flow-related enhancement" and results in an image with bright vessels on a dark background. It is important to emphasize that blood velocity is the major determinant of

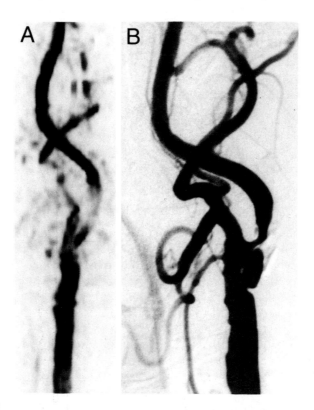

FIGURE 5.

A, magnetic resonance angiography study of a high-grade internal carotid stenosis. The vessel lumen is not well visualized because of low signal strength caused by disturbed flow at the site of stenosis. **B,** contrast arteriogram of the carotid bifurcation shown in **A.** The internal carotid lumen is severely stenotic, and a complex irregular plaque is demonstrated clearly.

signal strength in magnetic resonance angiography. In conventional arteriography, contrast material rapidly fills the vessel and visualization of the lumen is largely independent of hemodynamic patterns. The best magnetic resonance angiography images are obtained when the flow velocity is rapid and uniform across the arterial lumen. Areas of slow, disturbed, or turbulent flow may result in low signal strength and overestimation of stenosis on the study (Fig 5). This is especially likely to occur distal to a severe stenosis, where extreme turbulence causes complete loss of the signal, creating the appearance of an occlusion at the stenotic site. Another limitation of magnetic resonance imaging is the relatively long time required for acquisition of the signals used to produce the images. Since about 10 minutes may be needed to obtain an image, artifacts may be produced by swallowing or other patient movements during the acquisition period.

Experience with magnetic resonance angiography in the diagnosis of carotid artery disease is rather limited at present and few objective validation studies have been reported. In general, interpretation of these images has correlated closely with the results of contrast arteriography and duplex scanning.[29, 30] Problems have been encountered in identifying severe stenoses and occlusions due to the flow artifacts mentioned previously. It also has been difficult to assess the surface features of atherosclerotic plaque on magnetic resonance angiography images.

CLINICAL APPLICATIONS

The primary goal in the initial diagnostic evaluation of carotid artery disease is the identification of patients who are at risk for stroke. Once this is accomplished, decisions can be made regarding the need for arteriography and the potential benefits of carotid endarterectomy. Although attempts have been made to predict clinical outcome based on the B-mode image characteristics of carotid plaques, the degree of stenosis at the carotid bifurcation has been the most consistently reliable feature for assessing neurologic risk. Noninvasive tests provide a safe, cost-effective means for documenting the presence of carotid stenoses. The major indications for noninvasive testing are as follows: (1) an asymptomatic carotid bruit, (2) hemispheric cerebral or ocular transient ischemic attacks, (3) prior stroke with good neurologic recovery, (4) screening prior to major cardiac or peripheral vascular surgery, and (5) follow-up after carotid endarterectomy.[31] In the majority of cases, carotid duplex scanning is the preferred testing method and the only test necessary for screening or follow-up. Air-filled oculoplethysmography or transcranial Doppler may be indicated in selected patients to detect intracranial cerebrovascular disease or to assess collateral flow. These tests may be particularly useful when the duplex scan shows a relatively normal carotid bifurcation and atypical lesions are suspected. Other indirect noninvasive methods, such as the periorbital Doppler examination and fluid-filled oculoplethysmography, are not considered adequate for diagnostic use.

The finding of a bruit in the neck is one of the most common reasons for undertaking a noninvasive carotid evaluation. Among 100 patients with 165 asymptomatic bruits, duplex scanning showed a normal internal carotid in 12 (7%), less than 50% diameter stenosis in 83 (50%), a 50% or greater stenosis in 61 (37%), and internal carotid occlusion in 9 (6%).[32] Thus, although most neck bruits are associated with carotid disease, relatively few are related to severe internal carotid artery stenoses. Therapeutic decisions regarding patients with asymptomatic carotid disease must take into account not only the severity of stenosis, but also the expected clinical outcome. In a serial follow-up study of 167 patients with asymptomatic neck bruits, duplex scanning showed progression of disease in 60% of the internal carotid arteries.[33] The mean annual rate of progression to greater than 50% diameter stenosis was 8%, and the mean annual rate for development of ipsilateral neurologic symptoms (transient ischemic attack or stroke) was 4%. There was a strong correlation between the presence of an 80% to 99% internal carotid stenosis and the occurrence of neurologic symptoms or internal carotid occlusion. Patients with lesions of this severity had a 46% incidence of one or more of these events, whereas those with less severe stenoses had only a 1.5% incidence.

Although an asymptomatic 80% to 99% internal carotid stenosis appears to identify patients who are at high risk for neurologic symptoms or internal carotid occlusion, the clinically important question is whether this risk can be reduced by carotid endarterectomy. Although this question ultimately will be answered by randomized clinical trials, follow-up data are available on 129 asymptomatic 80% to 99% internal carotid stenoses, of which 56 were treated by carotid endarterectomy and 73 were followed without surgery.[34] There were no significant differences between patients who had undergone surgery and those who hadn't in characteristics such as age, diabetes mellitus, hypertension, ischemic heart disease, and aspirin use. During 24 months of follow-up, neurologic symptoms and internal carotid occlusion were significantly more frequent in the patients who hadn't undergone surgery (48%) than in those who had (9%). These results strongly suggest that endarterectomy improves the natural history of high-grade asymptomatic internal carotid stenoses, providing that the perioperative complication rate is extremely low. Follow-up studies also indicate that it is safe to follow asymptomatic patients with less than 80% internal carotid stenoses by duplex scanning at about 6-month intervals. If neurologic symptoms or progression to an 80% to 99% stenosis are observed, then the patient should be considered for carotid endarterectomy.

The purpose of screening in patients with hemispheric neurologic symptoms is to identify lesions that could reduce hemispheric blood flow or be the source of cerebral emboli. Although it generally is accepted that moderate carotid stenoses can be responsible for symptoms of cerebral ischemia, the most convincing data relate to severe stenoses. In the recently reported North American Symptomatic Carotid Endarterectomy Trial (NASCET), surgery was highly beneficial for patients with recent hemispheric transient ischemic attacks or mild strokes and 70% to 99% stenosis of the ipsilateral internal carotid artery.[35] Based on these results, symptomatic patients with severe carotid stenoses should be treated by endarterectomy unless their general medical condition makes the risk of surgery prohibitive. The optimal management of symptomatic patients with less than 70% carotid stenoses will remain uncertain until further data become available. Occasionally, the duplex scan shows a normal or minimally diseased internal carotid artery in a patient with neurologic symptoms. Follow-up of these patients generally supports a nonoperative approach, since the incidence of subsequent neurologic events is extremely low, and a noncarotid cause for symptoms may exist.[36]

The role of screening for carotid artery disease prior to cardiac or major peripheral vascular surgery is difficult to define. Studies that have reviewed this issue have not shown a consistent relationship between perioperative neurologic events and the presence of asymptomatic carotid stenoses.[37] Consequently, routine prophylactic carotid endarterectomy cannot be recommended. As noted previously, severe asymptomatic internal carotid stenoses are associated with an increased risk of neurologic symptoms and carotid occlusion. Therefore, if endarterectomy is indicated for asymptomatic carotid stenosis, this may take precedence over other elective surgical procedures.

Follow-up of patients after carotid endarterectomy with duplex scanning has documented the incidence and clinical significance of recurrent carotid stenoses. Symptomatic recurrent stenosis occurs in only about 5% of patients; however, the overall incidence is in the range of 9% to 21%.[38, 39] Serial duplex scanning also indicates that recurrent lesions tend to occur during the first 2 postoperative years, are tapered smoothly, and may regress over time. Recurrent lesions that persist generally remain stable, and progression to internal carotid occlusion is extremely rare. Since the incidence of neurologic symptoms does not appear to be significantly different in those patients with and without recurrent stenosis, a conservative approach to asymptomatic recurrent stenosis is justified.

Although noninvasive tests are used most commonly to screen patients for carotid artery disease, clinicians have relied on the results of computerized cerebral tomography to determine the optimal timing of carotid endarterectomy. Initial experience with carotid endarterectomy indicated that a delay of 4 to 6 weeks after an acute stroke was necessary to prevent the development of a hemorrhagic infarct.[40] However, the early reports appeared before computerized cerebral tomography was available and included patients with severe neurologic deficits and internal carotid occlusions who would not be considered good surgical candidates in the modern era. Subsequent experience suggests that patients with minor strokes and good neurologic recovery can undergo carotid endarterectomy safely without an arbitrary 4- to 6-week delay.[41]

It now appears that the presence of an infarct on computerized cerebral tomography in a patient with a stable, fixed neurologic deficit does not increase the risk of stroke related to elective carotid endarterectomy.[27, 42] In contrast, patients with acute neurologic deficits and infarcts on computerized cerebral tomography who undergo urgent carotid endarterectomy are at increased risk for neurologic morbidity and mortality.[42] Thus, routine computerized cerebral tomography in all patients being evaluated for carotid endarterectomy is not clinically indicated or cost effective.[43] However, computerized cerebral tomography can be helpful in planning treatment for patients with acute neurologic deficits and corresponding extracranial carotid lesions.

The use of magnetic resonance angiography in the diagnostic evaluation of carotid disease has several potential advantages over both duplex scanning and contrast arteriography. As discussed previously, magnetic resonance techniques can detect arterial lesions and evaluate the surrounding soft tissues with a single examination. It is likely that the ability of magnetic resonance angiography to image severe stenoses and occlusions will improve with further advances in technology. One unique aspect of magnetic resonance angiography is the possibility of obtaining full three-dimensional images of the carotid arteries. Although magnetic resonance angiography is noninvasive, it costs considerably more than carotid duplex scanning. Thus, its clinical use is justified only if it has distinct advantages over other established methods. Because of its limitations, magnetic resonance imaging is not an acceptable substitute for conventional arteriography at the present time, and duplex scanning remains the most cost-effective test for screening and follow-up studies.

In spite of the inherent high cost and risk, arteriography continues to be regarded as the definitive diagnostic test for identifying patients who are candidates for carotid endarterectomy. However, with improvements in the accuracy and reliability of carotid duplex scanning there has been increasing interest in performing carotid endarterectomy based on the clinical evaluation and duplex findings alone. Carotid bifurcation lesions that are suitable for endarterectomy include high-grade stenoses in asymptomatic patients and moderate to severe stenoses in patients with hemispheric neurologic symptoms; these are categories of lesions that can be detected accurately by duplex scanning. It often is emphasized that duplex scanning does not provide any direct information on lesions involving the proximal aortic arch branches or the intracranial circulation. However, clinical experience has shown that significant lesions proximal or distal to the carotid bifurcation are uncommon and rarely have an adverse effect on the outcome of carotid endarterectomy.[44] In addition, most stenoses in the proximal brachiocephalic vessels can be suspected on the basis of common carotid flow abnormalities or unequal arm blood pressures. Although the specific indications for carotid surgery without arteriography remain controversial, it has been shown that the results of arteriography rarely influence clinical decisions when a technically adequate duplex scan shows an ipsilateral 50% to 99% stenosis in a patient with hemispheric neurologic symptoms or an 80% to 99% stenosis in an asymptomatic patient.[45] Arteriography is most likely to be of value when the duplex scan is technically inadequate, for atypical lesions that appear to extend beyond the carotid bifurcation, and for less than 50% internal carotid stenoses in patients with neurologic symptoms. It seems inevitable that the tendency to perform more carotid surgery without contrast arteriography will increase as the technology of noninvasive testing continues to improve.

A suggested algorithm for the management of carotid artery disease based on noninvasive screening with duplex scanning is given in Figure 6. Like most such schemes, it provides general guidelines but does not account for all possible clinical circumstances. The suggested follow-up intervals are for a duplex scan to detect progressive or recurrent disease. Decisions to proceed with carotid endarterectomy assume that patients are medically fit for surgery. Because it occasionally is difficult to iden-

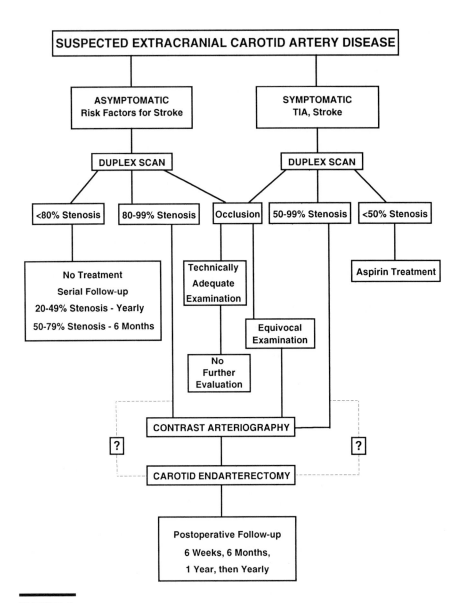

FIGURE 6.

Management algorithm for symptomatic and asymptomatic carotid disease based on noninvasive screening with duplex scanning. *TIA* = transient ischemic attack.

tify internal carotid occlusions by duplex scanning, equivocal examinations should be confirmed by arteriography if the patient is otherwise a surgical candidate. Although the specific NASCET criteria for carotid endarterectomy in symptomatic patients require a 70% to 99% stenosis by arteriography, most of the lesions in the 50% to 99% stenosis category by duplex scanning will fall into this group. Thus, the finding of a 50% to 99% carotid lesion in a symptomatic patient should be considered an indication for further evaluation. The option of proceeding directly to carotid endarterectomy based on the duplex scan results alone is indicated by the dotted lines in Figure 6.

REFERENCES

1. Moniz E: L'encephalographie arteriel, son importance dans la localisation des tumeurs cerebrales. Rev Neurol (Paris) 1927; 2:72–90.
2. Strandness DE Jr: Historical aspects, in Duplex Scanning in Vascular Disorders. New York, Raven Press, 1990, pp 1–24.
3. Bandyk DF, Thiele BL: Noninvasive assessment of carotid artery disease. West J Med 1983; 139:486–501.
4. Lye CR, Sumner DS, Strandness DE: The accuracy of the supraorbital Doppler examination in the diagnosis of hemodynamically significant carotid disease. Surgery 1976; 79:42–45.
5. Kartchner MM, McRae LP, Morrison FD: Noninvasive detection and evaluation of carotid occlusive disease. Arch Surg 1973; 106:528–535.
6. Gee W, Mehigan JT, Wylie EJ: Measurement of collateral hemispheric blood pressure by ocular pneumoplethysmography. Am J Surg 1975; 130:121–127.
7. Comerota AJ, Cranley JJ, Katz AK, et al: Real-time B-mode carotid imaging: A three-year multicenter experience. J Vasc Surg 1984; 1:84–95.
8. Hennerici M, Reifschneider G, Trockel U, et al: Detection of early atherosclerotic lesions by duplex scanning of the carotid artery. J Clin Ultrasound 1984; 12:455–464.
9. O'Donnell TF, Erdoes L, Mackay WC, et al: Correlation of B-mode ultrasound imaging and arteriography with pathologic findings at carotid endarterectomy. Arch Surg 1985; 120:443–449.
10. Reilly LM, Lusby RJ, Hughes L, et al: Carotid plaque histology using real-time ultrasonography—clinical and therapeutic implications. Am J Surg 1983; 146:188–193.
11. Lusby RJ, Ferell LD, Ehrenfeld WK, et al: Carotid plaque hemorrhage. Arch Surg 1981; 117:1479–1487.
12. O'Leary DH, Holen J, Ricotta JJ, et al: Carotid bifurcation disease—prediction of ulceration with B-mode US. Radiology 1987; 162:523–535.
13. Fell G, Phillips DJ, Chikos PM, et al: Ultrasonic duplex scanning for disease of the carotid artery. Circulation 1981; 64:1191–1195.
14. Langlois YE, Roederer GO, Chan AW, et al: Evaluating carotid artery disease—the concordance between pulsed Doppler/spectrum analysis and angiography. Ultrasound Med Biol 1983; 9:51–63.
15. Roederer GO, Langlois YE, Chan AW, et al: Ultrasonic duplex scanning of extracranial arteries: Improved accuracy using new features from the common carotid artery. J Cardiovasc Ultasonography 1982; 1:373–379.
16. Kohler T, Langlois Y, Roederer GO, et al: Sources of variability in carotid duplex examination: A prospective study. Ultrasound Med Biol 1985; 4:571–576.
17. Chikos PM, Fisher LD, Hirsh JA, et al: Observer variability in evaluating extracranial carotid artery stenosis. Stroke 1983; 14:885–892.
18. Zierler RE, Phillips DJ, Beach KW, et al: Noninvasive assessment of normal carotid bifurcation hemodynamics with color-flow ultrasound imaging. Ultrasound Med Biol 1987; 13:471–476.
19. Aaslid R, Markwalder TM, Nornes H: Non-invasive Doppler ultrasound recording of flow velocity in basal cerebral arteries. Neurosurgery 1982; 57:769–774.
20. DeWitt LD, Wechsler LR: Transcranial Doppler. Stroke 1988; 19:915–921.
21. Schneider PA, Rossman ME, Torem S, et al: Transcranial Doppler in the management of extracranial cerebrovascular disease: Implications in diagnosis and monitoring. J Vasc Surg 1988; 7:223–231.
22. Spencer MP, Thomas GI, Nicholls SC, et al: Detection of middle cerebral ar-

tery emboli during carotid endarterectomy using transcranial Doppler ultrasonography. *Stroke* 1990; 21:415–423.

23. Earnest F, Forbes G, Sandok BA, et al: Complications of cerebral angiography: Prospective assessment of risk. *AJNR* 1983; 4:1191–1197.

24. Martin-Paredero V, Dixon SM, Baker JD, et al: Risk of renal failure after major angiography. *Arch Surg* 1983; 118:1417–1420.

25. Russel JB, Watson TM, Modi JR, et al: Digital subtraction angiography for evaluation of extracranial carotid occlusive disease. Comparison with conventional arteriography. *Surgery* 1983; 97:604–611.

26. Eikelboom BC, Ackerstaff RGA, Ludwig JW, et al: Digital video subtraction angiography and duplex scanning in assessment of carotid artery disease: Comparison with conventional arteriography. *Surgery* 1983; 94:821–825.

27. Street DL, O'Brien MS, Ricotta JJ, et al: Observations on cerebral computed tomography in patients having carotid endarterectomy. *J Vasc Surg* 1988; 7:798–801.

28. Tsuruda JS, Saloner D, Anderson C: Noninvasive evaluation of cerebral ischemia—trends for the 1990s. *Circulation* 1991; 83(suppl I):176–189.

29. Ross JS, Masaryk TJ, Modic MT, et al: Magnetic resonance angiography of the extracranial carotid arteries and intracranial vessels: A review. *Neurology* 1989; 39:1369–1376.

30. Wilkerson DK, Keller I, Mezrich R, et al: The comparative evaluation of three-dimensional magnetic resonance for carotid artery disease. *J Vasc Surg* 1991; 14:803–811.

31. Strandness DE Jr, Andros G, Baker JD, et al: Vascular laboratory utilization and payment: Report of the ad hoc committee of the Western Vascular Society. *J Vasc Surg* 1992; 16:163–170.

32. Fell G, Breslau P, Knox RA, et al: Importance of noninvasive ultrasonic Doppler testing in the evaluation of patients with asymptomatic carotid bruits. *Am Heart J* 1981; 102:221–226.

33. Roederer GO, Langlois YE, Jager KA, et al: The natural history of carotid arterial disease in asymptomatic patients with cervical bruits. *Stroke* 1984; 15:605–613.

34. Moneta GL, Taylor DC, Nicholls SC, et al: Operative versus nonoperative management of asymptomatic high-grade internal carotid artery stenosis: Improved results with endarterectomy. *Stroke* 1987; 18:1005–1010.

35. North American Symptomatic Carotid Endarterectomy Trial Collaborators: Beneficial effect of carotid endarterectomy in symptomatic patients with high-grade carotid stenosis. *N Engl J Med* 1991; 325:445–453.

36. Zierler RE, Kohler TR, Strandness DE Jr: Duplex scanning of normal or minimally diseased carotid arteries: Correlation of arteriography and clinical outcome. *J Vasc Surg* 1990; 12:447–455.

37. Barnes RW, Liebman PR, Marszalek PB, et al: The natural history of asymptomatic carotid disease in patients undergoing cardiovascular surgery. *Surgery* 1981; 90:1075–1083.

38. Healy DA, Zierler RE, Nicholls SC, et al: Long-term follow-up and clinical outcome of carotid restenosis. *J Vasc Surg* 1989; 10:662–669.

39. Bernstein EF, Torem S, Dilley RB: Does carotid restenosis predict an increased risk of late symptoms, stroke, or death? *Ann Surg* 1990; 212:629–636.

40. Wylie EJ, Hein MF, Adams JE: Intracranial hemorrhage following surgical revascularization for treatment of acute strokes. *J Neurosurg* 1964; 21:212–215.

41. Piotrowski JJ, Bernhard VM, Rubin JR, et al: Timing of carotid endarterectomy after acute stroke. *J Vasc Surg* 1990; 11:45–52.

42. Ricotta JJ, Ouriel K, Green RM, et al: Use of computerized cerebral tomogra-

phy in selection of patients for elective and urgent carotid endarectomy. *Ann Surg* 1985; 202:783–787.

43. Martin JD, Valentine J, Myers SI, et al: Is routine CT scanning necessary in the preoperative evaluation of patients undergoing carotid endarterectomy? *J Vasc Surg* 1991; 14:267–270.

44. Roederer GO, Langlois YE, Chan ARW, et al: Is siphon disease important in predicting outcome of carotid endarterectomy. *Arch Surg* 1983; 118:1177–1181.

45. Dawson DL, Zierler RE, Kohler TR: Role of arteriography in the preoperative evaluation of carotid artery disease. *Am J Surg* 1991; 161:619–624.

PART II

Aortic Disease

Retroperitoneal Approach for Aortic Reconstruction

CALVIN B. ERNST, M.D.

ALEXANDER D. SHEPARD, M.D.

Before the modern era of abdominal aortic reconstruction, which arguably began in France with the first successful aortoiliac bypass for occlusive disease by Jacques Oudot on November 14, 1950[1] and with the first successful repair of an abdominal aortic aneurysm (AAA) by Charles Dubost on March 29, 1951,[2] the abdominal aorta and iliac arteries were exposed mainly for ligation procedures. In the late 18th century, John Abernethy used an extraperitoneal approach to ligate the external iliac artery.[3] In the early 19th century, Sir Astley Cooper used a similar approach to ligate the external iliac artery,[4] establishing the Abernethy-Cooper suprainguinal exposure of the external iliac vessels that continues to be used today.[5] These limited extraperitoneal exposures were extended by René Leriche, who, on July 24, 1939, resected the aortic bifurcation through the left retroperitoneum.[6] Leriche's goal was to relieve symptoms of aortoiliac occlusion by arterectomy and lumbar sympathectomy. As surgeons recognized the value of lumbar sympathectomy for managing occlusive arterial disease, other retroperitoneal exposures were described. It was not long after Leriche's report that Gordon Murray used the retroperitoneal approach to expose the aorta for embolectomy.[7] Thus, the evolution of the retroperitoneal approach to the abdominal aorta for reconstruction must be credited to several surgeons, eventuating in Oudot's and Dubost's seminal achievements.

Since these two landmark operations, aortic reconstruction has become safe and widely practiced, with almost 70,000 such operations performed in 1985.[8] However, retroperitoneal aortic exposure has not been adopted widely, probably because, as a result of training, general and vascular surgeons feel more comfortable working in the abdomen. Nonetheless, over the past 3 decades, refinements by Rob, Schumacker, Williams, and other surgeons have established the value of this retroperitoneal aortic reconstruction, particularly for certain patients and under specific circumstances.[9–21]

This chapter will review the indications, technique, and results of retroperitoneal aortic reconstruction for AAAs, aortoiliac occlusive disease (AIOD), and other complex aortic lesions.

Advances in Vascular Surgery, vol. 1.
©1993, Mosby–Year Book, Inc.

ADVANTAGES AND DISADVANTAGES

Several investigators have compared retroperitoneal to transperitoneal aortic reconstruction and cite several advantages of the former over the latter.[14, 17–19] All of these reports were retrospective reviews, however. Most studies include patients with AIOD and AAA. One retrospective study describing aortic reconstruction for AIOD notes better results with retroperitoneal than transperitoneal exposure. This same report, however, states that AAA is a contraindication to the retroperitoneal approach.[22] In another study, the authors concluded that complex aortic reconstruction for AAA was facilitated through the retroperitoneal approach.[23] The only prospective randomized study comparing transperitoneal and retroperitoneal aortic exposure concluded that there was no important advantage or physiologic superiority of retroperitoneal over transperitoneal aortic repair.[20]

Such conflicting data present a dilemma as to which approach is better. It has been suggested that retroperitoneal aortic reconstruction, for both AAA and AIOD, is less stressful to the patient, with less postoperative ileus, less operative evaporative fluid loss, less third-space fluid shifts, lower blood transfusion requirements, and fewer pulmonary complications than transperitoneal aortic reconstruction. Consequently, the retroperitoneal approach has been recommended for elderly and medically high-risk patients, and for those with complex aortic disease. However, until additional prospective data are available comparing transperitoneal and retroperitoneal aortic reconstruction, no definitive conclusions can be drawn favoring either approach.

Disadvantages of the retroperitoneal approach include inability to examine intra-abdominal organs thoroughly, inaccessibility of all but the proximal 1 cm of the right renal artery, and relative inaccessibility of the right external iliac artery.

INDICATIONS AND CONTRAINDICATIONS

In spite of conflicting opinions, for selected patients, retroperitoneal aortic exposure appears superior to transperitoneal exposure. In some, it is because of the extent and anatomy of aortic disease; in others, it is because extra-aortic pathology precludes safe transperitoneal aortic reconstruction.

Indications for retroperitoneal aortic reconstruction include patients with morbid obesity, horseshoe kidney, and abdominal wall ostomies. It also is indicated for patients who have extensive intra-abdominal adhesions (hostile abdomen) resulting from previous abdominal operations, radiation therapy, or inflammatory processes. Complex aortic problems facilitated by the retroperitoneal approach include large AAA (greater than 10 cm); suprarenal or juxtarenal AAA; aortic pathology requiring adjunctive left renal, celiac, or superior mesenteric artery (SMA) reconstruction; secondary aortic procedures, and inflammatory AAA. Some even have recommended the retroperitoneal approach for ruptured AAAs.[24] However, experience is required in elective retroperitoneal AAA repair before using this approach for ruptured AAA. Since few surgeons outside major medical centers have experience with retroperitoneal aortic reconstruction, its use in the management of ruptured AAA is questioned seriously.

The only absolute contraindication to retroperitoneal aortic reconstruction is the need to perform an adjunctive right aortorenal bypass. Relative contraindications include the need to use the right external iliac artery for aortoiliac bypass, ruptured AAA, and the need to examine intra-abdominal organs thoroughly.

PREOPERATIVE EVALUATION

Beyond the standard preoperative evaluation and preparation employed for any patient undergoing aortic reconstruction for aneurysmal or occlusive disease, no special studies are required when use of the retroperitoneal approach is anticipated. Comorbid conditions, particularly cardiac disease and others that may add to the morbidity and mortality of aortic reconstruction, must be addressed thoroughly.

In a comprehensive analysis of 1,000 patients undergoing peripheral vascular operations, including 263 patients with AAAs, Hertzer identified severe correctable coronary artery disease in 31% of those with AAAs.[25] Of note was that surgical coronary artery disease was present in 41% of those suspected of having it by clinical criteria and in 18% of those without clinical suspicion for coronary artery disease. Furthermore, since cardiac disease is the most common cause of death following aortic reconstruction, a thorough cardiac evaluation is required. Depending on the patient's ability to exercise, such evaluation will include exercise stress echocardiography or exercise stress thallium 201 cardiac imaging. If the patient is unable to exercise, dipyridamole thallium 201 cardiac imaging has proven to be reliable for selecting those who require coronary arteriography and possible myocardial revascularization prior to aortic reconstruction. Additional nonexercise stress tests include two-dimensional echocardiography, multigaited ejection fraction scintigraphy, and dobutamine stress echocardiography.

Although ischemic myocardial events are the leading causes for morbidity and mortality among patients undergoing aortic reconstruction, other comorbidities must be identified and corrected as well. These include pulmonary and renal diseases. Spirometric tests can identify and quantitate both obstructive and restrictive pulmonary disease effectively. Marginal pulmonary function, particularly a vital capacity and 1-second forced expiratory volume of less than 50% of predicted, suggests significant pulmonary compromise. Maximum voluntary ventilation measures both airway resistance and ventilatory function, and a value less than 50% of predicted confirms significant pulmonary compromise. Such pulmonary disease should be treated preoperatively, especially if lower left thoracotomy is an anticipated part of the retroperitoneal procedure. Marginal renal function reflected by serum creatinine elevations over 1.8 mg/dL must be evaluated and corrected, if possible. Of particular note is that ischemic nephropathy associated with occlusive renal artery disease may respond favorably to adjunctive renal revascularization during aortic reconstruction.[26]

OPERATIVE TECHNIQUE

POSITIONING

Depending upon the segment of aorta requiring exposure (infrarenal, juxtarenal, suprarenal) and the type of incision to be used (extended left flank, transverse abdominal), the patient lies supine or is turned into the right lateral decubitus position with the left thorax elevated 45 to 60 degrees. We prefer the latter position because it provides greater versatility and ability to expose the juxtarenal and supraceliac aorta than does supine positioning. With the left thorax up, the hips should lie as flat as possible to provide access to both groins. The patient is placed on an air-vacuum styrofoam bean bag, the table is jackknifed, and the bag is evacuated to maintain the patient's position (Fig 1). The flexion point of the table should be midway between the right costal margin and the right iliac crest. With the patient secured to the table by the bean bag and the left arm positioned across the thorax and secured to an armrest, the table may be rotated to the right during aortic dissection or to the left during right groin dissection. The table is flattened during wound closure to bring the incision edges into apposition.

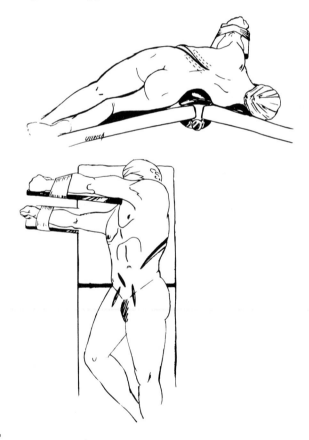

FIGURE 1.

Position of patient and placement of incision for extended left flank retroperitoneal aortic exposure. (From Shepard AD, Scott GR, Mackey WC, et al: *Arch Surg* 1986; 121:445. Used by permission.)

INCISION

Several descriptions of retroperitoneal aortic exposure have been provided using transverse, midline, or paramedian incisions.[9, 10, 27] For infrarenal aortic exposure, we prefer an oblique incision beginning at the lateral margin of the left rectus sheath midway between the symphysis pubis and umbilicus, and extending laterally into the 11th intercostal space.[23, 28] When exposing the supraceliac or pararenal aorta, the incision extends into the 9th or 10th intercostal space. With the 11th interspace incision, the left chest is not entered and a short segment of 12th rib is excised to facilitate later closure. When entering the 9th or 10th intercostal spaces, the diaphragm is incised either radially or circumferentially for a short distance, but not down to the aortic hiatus, to prevent tearing the costal attachments of the diaphragm when spreading the ribs.

AORTIC EXPOSURE

The retroperitoneal space is entered at the tip of the 12th rib and, with blunt dissection, the peritoneum is stripped away from the underlying transversalis fascia anteriorly and the lumbodorsal fascia posteriorly. As the peritoneum is dissected from the abdominal wall at the linea semilunaris, care is taken to avoid tearing the peritoneum, which is thin and adherent at this site. For most aortic procedures, the retrorenal plane is dissected and the left kidney and ureter are mobilized and retracted anteriorly and to the right (Fig 2). Alternatively, the left kidney may remain

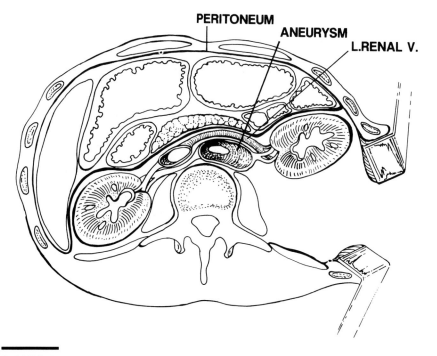

FIGURE 2.

Cross-sectional diagram of the abdomen demonstrating the retrorenal approach used for most aortic reconstructive procedures. The left *(L)* renal vein *(V)* does not obscure the juxtarenal aorta.

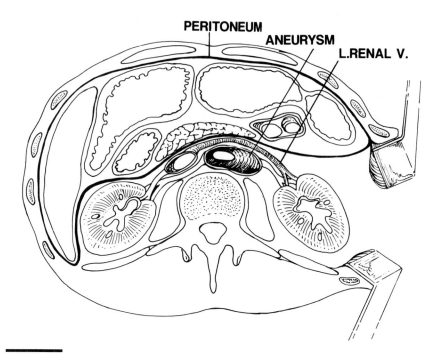

PERITONEUM

ANEURYSM

L.RENAL V.

FIGURE 3.

Cross-sectional diagram of the abdomen demonstrating the approach anterior to the left kidney that is necessary for exposure of the proximal superior mesenteric artery. L = left; V = vein.

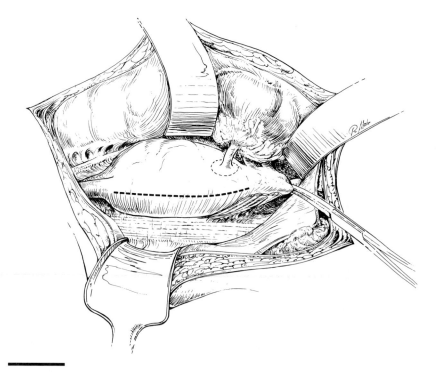

FIGURE 4.

Exposure of a suprarenal abdominal aortic aneurysm through the extended left flank retroperitoneal approach. Note that limited dissection is required for placement of the supraceliac aortic clamp. (From Shepard AD, Tollefson DFJ, Reddy DJ, et al: *J Vasc Surg* 1991; 14:286. Used by permission.)

in situ, but under these circumstances, the left renal vein obscures the juxtarenal aorta (Fig 3).

Exposure of the suprarenal and supraceliac aorta requires mobilization of the pancreas along with the left kidney. The diaphragmatic crus enveloping the aorta is divided with electrocautery and the paraceliac aorta is dissected. Suture ligation of periaortic areolar tissue at the level of the SMA and celiac origins minimizes lymphatic leaks. Exposure of the proximal several centimeters of the SMA requires leaving the left kidney in situ. Circumferential dissection of the supraceliac or infrarenal aortic segments is not required for proximal aortic clamping. Only narrow tunnels to accommodate the blades of a vascular clamp anterior and posterior to the aorta are made (Fig 4).

DISTAL EXPOSURE

Exposure of the full length of the left iliac artery and proximal right common iliac artery is obtained easily, but exposure of the right iliac bifurcation and distal right external iliac artery is not possible unless the patient is very thin. If exposure of this area is required, a small right lower quadrant extraperitoneal incision is made and the right external iliac artery is approached extraperitoneally. Rotating the table to the left, toward the surgeon, facilitates right external iliac or right femoral artery dissection. The proximal right common iliac artery must be dissected cautiously, because injury to the inferior vena cava at this site is hazardous and difficult to control. Therefore, intraluminal balloon occlusion of the right iliac arterial system often is favored over mobilization of the iliac artery for clamp occlusion. This is particularly true when managing a large AAA where the right common iliac artery may be obscured. Some have recommended extending the abdominal incision across the midline into the right lower quadrant to facilitate right iliac artery exposure, but the peritoneal cavity often is entered with this maneuver.

When using retroperitoneal exposure to manage AIOD, aortic mobilization is limited to a 5- to 6-cm infrarenal segment. Under these circumstances, the inferior mesenteric artery (IMA) may be in the way, since the left colon has been mobilized up and to the right. Although division of the IMA improves exposure, in most situations, the IMA should be left intact to allow retrograde perfusion through the aortofemoral bypass graft. When managing an aneurysm confined to the aorta, the aneurysm is opened behind the IMA ostium. If IMA reconstruction is not required, the IMA ostium is oversewn from inside the opened aneurysm. If necessary, a Carrel patch of IMA can be implanted into the body of the prosthesis or the left graft limb. Occasionally, when managing a large AAA, the IMA impedes access to the right iliac vessels and it can be divided flush with the aneurysm. If IMA reconstruction is anticipated, a small bulldog clamp is used to occlude the IMA temporarily during aortic grafting.

AORTIC CLAMP PLACEMENT

When managing a juxtarenal AAA with the aortic clamp at either the suprarenal or supraceliac levels, back bleeding from the right renal artery

TABLE 1.

Retroperitoneal vs. Transperitoneal Aortic Reconstruction*

Author	Number		Postoperative Ventilation		Postoperative Ileus (days)		ICU Stay (days)	
	TP	RP	TP	RP	TP	RP	TP	RP
Peck et al. (1986)	70	200	NS	NS	4	2	2	1
Sicard et al. (1987)	50	54	0.8 days	1.0 day	4.0	2.4	2.0	2.1
Leather et al. (1989)	106	193	3.2 days	1.3 days	2.7	0.3	4.0	1.4
Cambria et al.† (1990)	59	54	5.1 hr	2.6 hr	4.0	3.4	NS, but no difference	
Shepard et al. (1991)	30	17	1.2 days	1.0 day	3.4	2.9	3.6	2.8

*ICU = intensive care unit; TP = transperitoneal; RP = retroperitoneal; NS = not stated.
†Only prospective randomized study.
‡Based on 60 abdominal aortic aneurysms repaired in standard fashion; others treated by exclusion/bypass.

may be controlled with a small balloon occlusion catheter and that from the left renal artery with a small bulldog clamp. Back bleeding from the SMA, celiac, and lumbar arteries is controlled by an aortic balloon occlusion catheter. For minimal back bleeding, however, the operative field is kept dry by using the autotransfusor suction. After the proximal anastomosis is completed, an atraumatic padded clamp is placed across the prosthesis and the aortic clamp is removed, restoring renal and visceral blood flow.

We feel that it is safer and easier to clamp the supraceliac aorta than the suprarenal aorta, particularly when extensive atherosclerotic plaque involves the posterior aspect of the aorta at the level of the renal arteries and SMA. Supraceliac occlusion is well tolerated for the brief time required to complete the proximal anastomosis.[23, 29, 30]

When clamping the aorta at any level, cardiac function is monitored carefully. Optimal cardiac output is maintained by volume loading and the use of sodium nitroprusside to decrease afterload and left ventricular work. Mannitol is administered before aortic clamping to maintain a brisk diuresis. Heparin sodium is not given or is given in low dosage when supraceliac clamping is employed, because of the coagulopathy frequently associated with temporary visceral ischemia. Cold renal perfusion (250 mL per kidney) consisting of 500 mL of 4° C Ringer's lactate solution containing 12.5 g of mannitol, 1,000 units of heparin sodium, and 44 mEq of $NaHCO_3$ is used selectively with suprarenal or supraceliac clamping. It usually is reserved for patients with renal dysfunction (serum creatinine $\geq$ 1.8 mg/dL) or for those in whom prolonged ($>$ 30 to 40 minutes) renal ischemia is anticipated.

Hospital Stay (days)		Estimated Blood Loss (mL)		Operative Mortality (%)		Morbidy (number of patients)		Wound Problems (%)	
TP	RP	TP	RP	TP	RP	TP	RP	TP	RP
10	7	NS	NS	3	1.5	53/70	55/200	1.4	1.5
14	10	1,950	1,296	2	1.9	16/50	8/54	4.0	4.6
12	7	1,756	1,321‡	3.8	3.6	28/106	21/193	0.0	1.0
9.5	9.3	921	910	1.7	0.0	19/59	16/54	5.0	4.0
10.7	8.1	2,136	1,577	0.0	0.0	NS	NS	NS	NS

WOUND CLOSURE

Wound closure is straightforward and is facilitated by flattening the operating table. The retroperitoneum is not drained, but meticulous electrocautery hemostasis is obtained, since many small vessels tend to ooze following retroperitoneal dissection. If the chest has been entered, the diaphragm is closed around a catheter, which is removed after the evacuation of pleural air and expansion of the lung.

RESULTS

Most reports of retroperitoneal aortic reconstruction have been based upon retrospective analyses. Nonetheless, the majority of authors reporting on retroperitoneal aortic reconstruction describe advantages over the transperitoneal approach (Table 1). However, most studies are not comparable. For example, Sicard and his colleagues, and Cambria and his coworkers described a limited anterolateral approach to the infrarenal aorta,[18, 20] whereas other authors use a more extensive dissection and posterolateral approach to the aorta for complex aortic lesions.[11, 15, 19, 23] Although claims are made favoring retroperitoneal aortic reconstruction over the standard transperitoneal approach, only one prospective randomized study has been reported. It concluded that there is ". . . no physiologic superiority for the retroperitoneal approach and thus no support for its routine adoption as the preferred technique . . ."[20] Most authors agree with this conclusion, but certain advantages favor the retroperitoneal approach for aortic reconstruction (Table 2).

TABLE 2.

Advantages of Retroperitoneal Aortic Exposure

Avoids scarring/adhesions from previous intra-abdominal operations
Simplifies proximal abdominal aortic exposure and control
Improves exposure of aneurysm neck with large abdominal aortic
  aneurysms
Easier aortic exposure in the obese patient
Avoids hemodynamic problems associated with mesenteric traction
Decreases postoperative ileus
Decreases postoperative respiratory morbidity
Faster, smoother postoperative recovery

Of 581 patients undergoing aortic reconstructive procedures at the Henry Ford Hospital between 1985 and 1990, 114 (21%) have been performed using the left retroperitoneal approach.[12] For complex aortic lesions requiring supraceliac aortic clamping, results have been excellent. Using this approach in 85 patients, 70 of whom had AAAs and 50% of whom required suprarenal or supraceliac aortic clamping, the operative mortality rate for elective procedures was 1.2%.[23] Postoperative recovery was rapid and similar to that of historic control patients undergoing straightforward transperitoneal infrarenal AAA repair.

One physiologic advantage of retroperitoneal over transperitoneal aortic reconstruction relates to avoidance of mesenteric prostacyclin release.[31] A decrease in mean arterial pressure and systemic vascular resistance, increase in cardiac index, and facial flushing following bowel manipulation and traction during transperitoneal aortic exposure was documented. These changes were not observed with the retroperitoneal approach. Beyond physiologic differences favoring the retroperitoneal approach, one must be aware of the disadvantages of retroperitoneal aortic exposure (Table 3).

Surgeons experienced with retroperitoneal aortic reconstruction recognized that certain pitfalls exist that, for the uninitiated, may condemn this procedure. However, these problems may be anticipated and avoided with alternative approaches to the aorta, including the standard transperitoneal approach and transperitoneal-retroperitoneal exposure, otherwise known as medial visceral rotation.

Certain pitfalls deserve comment, such as injury to the inferior vena

TABLE 3.

Disadvantages of Retroperitoneal Aortic Exposure

Limited exposure of right renal artery
Poor exposure of right iliac bifurcation
Unable to evaluate fully concomitant intra-abdominal disease
Requires more time for patient positioning

cava, which is very difficult to manage through left retroperitoneal exposure. Unrecognized splenic trauma may result from overly vigorous anterior retraction of the peritoneal sac under the left costal margin. It is necessary to identify the lumbar branch of the left renal vein, not only to avoid injury, but also because it serves as a marker of the origin of the left renal artery. Similarly, a retroaortic left renal vein may be injured if it is not recognized. The left gonadal vein must be identified when sweeping the retroperitoneal structures anteriorly so that it is not avulsed from the left renal vein. Also, the left ureter must be identified when mobilizing the retroperitoneal structures to avoid injury. During secondary aortic procedures, the left ureter is particularly vulnerable to traction injury because it may be tethered in the pelvis and not as mobile as during primary aortic reconstruction. The cecum may be tethered into the right iliac fossa as a result of previous appendectomy and may be vulnerable to injury in the event tunneling to the right groin is required. The left renal artery and IMA are mobilized anteriorly when retrorenal dissection is performed and both must be identified to avoid injury. The anteriorly displaced IMA may limit exposure of the right iliac vessels. Under such circumstances, the IMA should be divided and ligated flush with the aorta (if operating for AAA) to preserve collateral continuity from the superior mesenteric to the hypogastric circulations. Furthermore, it is important to open the AAA posterior to the IMA origin if one anticipates the need for IMA reconstruction. An unrecognized left pneumothorax may develop, particularly if the left intercostal incision is not made carefully. A precise intercostal incision with preservation of the intercostal nerves also will prevent postoperative weakness of the left abdominal musculature and troublesome left flank bulge with abdominal asymmetry that has been reported following use of the retroperitoneal approach.[32]

SUMMARY

The ability to expose the aorta by the retroperitoneal approach should be part of a vascular surgeon's repertoire, in spite of the fact that this approach is required in less than 25% of all patients undergoing aortic reconstruction. In particular, it is useful for complex aortic reconstructive procedures in high-risk patients. Knowledge of the pitfalls of and precise indications and contraindications for the procedure may preclude preventable complications of left retroperitoneal aortic exposure, thereby increasing the utility of this valuable approach.

REFERENCES

1. Oudot J: La greffe vascularies dans les thromboses due carrefour aortique. *Presse Med* 1951: 59:234–236.
2. Dubost C, Allary M, Oecunomos N: Resection of an aneurysm of the abdominal aorta: Reestablishment of the continuity by a preserved human arterial graft with result after five months. *Arch Surg* 1952; 64:405–408.
3. Abernethy J: *Surgical Observations*. London, Longman & Orees, 1804, pp 209–231.
4. Cooper A: Case of femoral aneurism for which the external iliac artery was

tied by Sir Astley Cooper, Bt. an account of the preparation of the limb, dissected at the expiration of eighteen years. Taken from Sir Astley Cooper's notes. *Guys Hosp Rep* 1836; 1:43–52.

5. Shumacker HB Jr: Extraperitoneal approach to vascular operations. *South Med J* 1982; 75:1499–1507.

6. Leriche R: De la résection due carrefour aorticoiliaque avec double sympathectomie lombaire pour thrombose artéritique de l'aorte. Le syndrome de l'oblitération termino-aortique par arterite. *Presse Med* 1940; 55:601–604.

7. Murray G: Aortic embolectomy. *Surg Gynecol Obstet* 1943; 97:157–162.

8. Ernst CB, Rutkow IM, Cleveland RJ, et al: Vascular surgery in the United States. Report of the Joint Society for Vascular Surgery-International Society for Cardiovascular Surgery Committee on Vascular Surgical Manpower. *J Vasc Surg* 1987; 7:611–621.

9. Rob C: Extraperitoneal approach to the abdominal aorta. *Surgery* 1963; 53:87–89.

10. Shumacker HB Jr: Midline extraperitoneal exposure of the abdominal aorta and iliac arteries. *Surg Gynecol Obstet* 1972; 135: 791–792.

11. Williams GM, Ricotta J, Zinner M, et al: The extended retroperitoneal approach for extensive atherosclerosis of the aorta and renal vessels. *Surgery* 1980; 88:846–855.

12. Stipa S, Shaw RS: Aorto-iliac reconstruction through a retroperitoneal approach. *J Cardiovasc Surg* 1968; 9:224–236.

13. Taheri SA, Nowakowski PA, Stoesser FG: Retroperitoneal approach to aortic surgery: Experiences with 75 consecutive cases. *Vasc Surg* 1969; 3:144–148.

14. Peck JJ:, McReynolds DG, Baker DH, et al: Extraperitoneal approach for aortoiliac reconstruction of the abdominal aorta. *Am J Surg* 1986; 151:620–623.

15. Shepard AD, Scott GR, Mackey WC, et al: Retroperitoneal approach to high-risk abdominal aortic aneurysms. *Arch Surg* 1986; 121:444–449.

16. Helsby R, Moosa AR: Aorto-iliac reconstruction with special reference to the extraperitoneal approach. *Br J Surg* 1975; 62:596–600.

17. Sicard GA, Freeman MB, VanderWoude JC, et al: Comparison between the transabdominal and retroperitoneal approach for reconstruction of the infrarenal abdominal aorta. *J Vasc Surg* 1987; 5:19–27.

18. Sicard GA, Allen BT, Munn JS, et al: Retroperitoneal versus transperitoneal approach for repair of abdominal aortic aneurysms. *Surg Clin North Am* 1989; 69:795–806.

19. Leather RP, Shah DM, Kaufman JL, et al: Comparative analysis of retroperitoneal and transperitoneal aortic replacement for aneurysm. *Surg Gynecol Obstet* 1989; 168:387–393.

20. Cambria RP, Brewster DC, Abbott WM, et al: Transperitoneal versus retroperitoneal approach for aortic reconstruction: A randomized prospective study. *J Vasc Surg* 1990; 11:314–325.

21. Shah DM, Chang BB, Paty PSK, et al: Treatment of abdominal aortic aneurysm by exclusion and bypass: An analysis of outcome. *J Vasc Surg* 1991; 13:15–22.

22. Johnson JN, McLoughlin GA, Wake PN, et al: Comparison of extraperitoneal and transperitoneal methods of aorto-iliac reconstruction. *J Cardiovasc Surg* 1986; 27:561–564.

23. Shepard AD, Tollefson DFJ, Reddy DJ, et al: Left flank peritoneal exposure: A technical aid to complex aortic reconstruction. *J Vasc Surg* 1991; 14:283–291.

24. Chang BB, Shah DM, Paty PSK, et al: Can the retroperitoneal approach be used for ruptured abdominal aortic aneurysms? *J Vasc Surg* 1990; 11:326–330.

25. Hertzer NR, Beven EG, Young JR, et al: Coronary artery disease in peripheral vascular patients. A classification of 1000 coronary angiograms and results of surgical management. *Ann Surg* 1984; 199:223–333.
26. Dean RH, Tribble RW, Hansen KJ, et al: Evolution of renal insufficiency in ischemic nephropathy. *Ann Surg* 1991; 213:446–456.
27. Taheri SA, Sawronski S, Smith D: Paramedian approach to the abdominal aorta. *J Cardiovasc Surg* 1983; 24:529–531.
28. Ernst CB: Retroperitoneal approach to the abdominal aorta, in Haimovici H, Callow AD, DePalma RG, et al (eds): *Vascular Surgery, Principles and Techniques.* Norwalk, Connecticut, Appleton & Lange, 1989, pp 245–250.
29. Green RM, Ricotta JJ, Ouriel K, et al: Results of supraceliac aortic clamping in the difficult elective resection of infrarenal abdominal aortic aneurysm. *J Vasc Surg* 1989; 9:124–134.
30. Nypaver TJ, Shepard AD, Reddy DJ, et al: Supraceliac aortic cross-clamping: Determinants of outcome in elective abdominal aortic reconstruction. *J Vasc Surg*, in press.
31. Hudson JC, Wurm WH, O'Donnell TF Jr, et al: Hemodynamics and prostacyclin release in the early phases of aortic surgery: Comparison of transabdominal and retroperitoneal approaches. *J Vasc Surg* 1988; 7:190–198.
32. Honig MP, Mason RA, Giron F: Wound complications of the retroperitoneal approach to the aorta and iliac vessels. *J Vasc Surg* 1992; 15:28–34.

Reducing the Risk of Spinal Cord Injury During Thoracoabdominal Aortic Aneurysm Repair

THOMAS C. NASLUND, M.D.

LARRY H. HOLLIER, M.D.

I schemic spinal cord injury with neurologic dysfunction has been re-ported to occur in 4% to 30% of patients undergoing repair of aneu-rysms of the thoracoabdominal aorta.[1, 2] Although multiple adjunctive measures have been used, no single intervention has prevented spinal cord injury. Using a multimodality protocol, however, we have recorded a low rate of spinal cord injury in recent years.

SPINAL CORD BLOOD SUPPLY

The spinal cord receives blood from the single anterior and paired pos-terior spinal arteries. Intraspinal communications between anterior and posterior spinal arteries do not exist and, thus, the anterior spinal artery supplies the anterior two thirds of the spinal cord (including the motor tracts) and the posterior spinal arteries supply the posterior one third of the spinal cord (dorsal columns, Fig 1). The anterior spinal artery blood supply arises from the basilar artery and radicular arteries arising from vertebral, costocervical trunk, upper and lower thoracic intercostal, and branches of the hypogastric arteries (Fig 2). Additionally, the anterior spi-nal artery receives blood from multiple radicular spinal arteries that arise as branches of intercostal arteries. The exact spinal level at which the ra-dicular arteries arise is variable, but the largest, commonly known as the artery of Adamkiewicz, usually arises as a branch of an intercostal artery between the T8 and L2 spinal levels.[3] The posterior spinal arteries re-ceive more numerous radicular branches; therefore, posterior spinal ar-tery flow less often is reduced critically during aortic surgery. Occlusion of the thoracic aorta reduces distal aortic pressure and, as a result, perfu-sion pressure in the thoracic intercostal and hypogastric arteries. In pa-tients with an intact anterior spinal artery, blood flow from the basilar

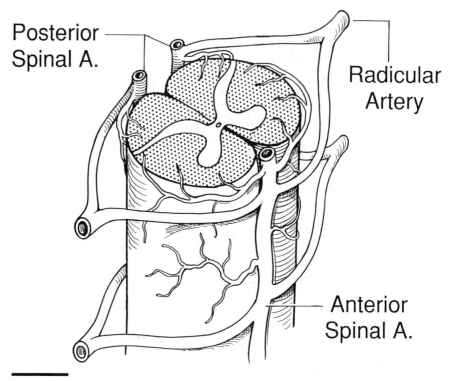

FIGURE 1.

Diagrammatic representation of spinal cord blood supply to anterior two thirds and posterior one third of the spinal cord. A = artery. (From Cohen JR (ed): *Vascular Surgery 2000*. Austin, RG Landis Co, 1991. Used by permission.)

arteries and other cephalad radicular arteries may prevent spinal cord ischemia. In many patients, however, the anterior spinal artery is not contiguous, and regions of the spinal cord (lower thoracic and lumbar) may be dependent on segmental sources of blood flow. In such situations, thoracic aortic clamping can render the lower thoracic and lumbar spinal cord ischemic.

PATHOPHYSIOLOGY OF ISCHEMIC SPINAL CORD INJURY

Complete understanding of the events that lead to neuronal death following ischemia has yet to be obtained, but some of the events that result in neuronal injury can be deduced and others can be ascertained from laboratory findings. Figure 3 provides a diagrammatic representation of events that lead to paraplegia after spinal cord ischemia and various interventions that can reduce the severity of neuronal insult at each point in the sequence of events.

CLINICAL MANIFESTATIONS OF SPINAL CORD ISCHEMIA

Neurologic outcome after thoracoabdominal aortic surgery cannot be predicted accurately in an individual patient because of variability in both

Human Spinal Blood Supply

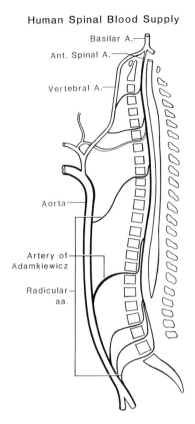

FIGURE 2.

Spinal cord radicular arteries (aa) supplying blood flow to the anterior spinal artery (A). (From Cohen JR (ed): *Vascular Surgery 2000.* Austin, RG Landis Co, 1991. Used by permission.)

the extent of the aneurysm and the blood supply to the spinal cord. It can be assumed that many, if not all, patients undergoing thoracoabdominal aortic surgery experience some degree of spinal cord ischemia. This likely is transient, and most patients recover fully after revascularization is complete. Any transient neurologic deficit that might occur in such situations may be masked by the fact that the patient is under general anesthesia.

Many patients who suffer neurologic deficits after thoracoabdominal aortic surgery present with acute-onset paraplegia. This neurologic deficit is noticed at the time the patient awakens from anesthesia and is characterized by flaccid paralysis of the lower extremities. Acute-onset paraplegia probably is induced from ischemia severe enough to cause early neuronal death. Clearly, inadequate revascularization of the spinal cord by exclusion of critical intercostal arteries could cause this type of deficit. Additionally, intercostal artery thrombosis, embolization, reperfusion injury, and acute spinal cord edema all could play a role. The severity of neurologic dysfunction can range from sphincter dysfunction caused by conus medullaris dysfunction, to paraparesis or dense paraplegia.

PARAPLEGIA

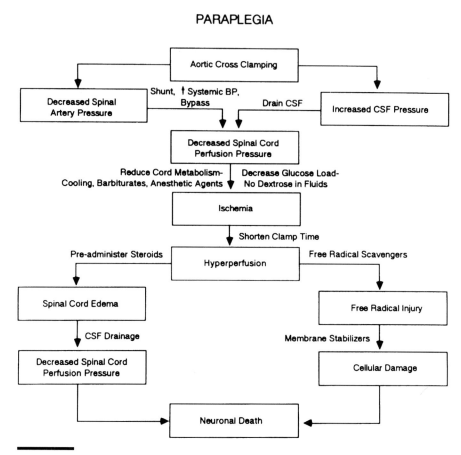

FIGURE 3.

Sequence of physiologic events following ischemia that lead to neuronal injury in the spinal cord. BP = blood pressure; CSF = cerebrospinal fluid. (From Moore W (ed): *Vascular Surgery: A Comprehensive Review*. Philidelphia, WB Saunders Co, 1991. Used by permission.)

Perhaps as many as 50% of the neurologic deficits that result from thoracoabdominal aortic surgery are of the delayed-onset variety.[1] Patients awaken from anesthesia entirely normal, then develop a deficit later. Again, the severity of the deficit is variable, but it has been our experience that these types of deficits usually involve paraparesis and develop between 1 and 9 days postoperatively. Since instituting a multimodality protocol designed to reduce the risk of spinal cord injury from ischemia, we have noticed a trend toward reduction in the incidence of acute-onset paraplegia but not delayed-onset paraplegia. We have attributed these observations to incomplete protection of the spinal cord sufficient to avoid acute-onset paraplegia, but not delayed-onset deficits. Such a hypothesis requires that delayed-onset deficits are induced by a lesser degree of ischemia than is needed to cause acute-onset deficits. This has been confirmed in the laboratory by observing that rabbits with spinal cord ischemia manifest acute-onset paraplegia with extensive aortic clamping and a high incidence of delayed-onset deficits with intermediate aortic clamping.[4]

The etiology of delayed-onset paraplegia remains elusive. It can be assumed, however, that the same pathophysiologic processes involved in the development of acute paraplegia also might be active in the development of delayed-onset paraplegia.

SPINAL CORD PROTECTION DURING OPERATION

Absolute prevention of paraplegia from thoracoabdominal aortic surgery is not yet possible. No single therapeutic intervention has been shown to protect the spinal cord from ischemic injury in all cases of thoracoabdominal aortic surgery. The risk of spinal cord injury has been reduced, however, using a multimodality perioperative protocol designed to (1) limit the severity of spinal cord ischemia, (2) reduce the metabolic rate of the ischemic spinal cord, and (3) limit reperfusion injury of the spinal cord.

Severity of ischemia is related in part to duration of clamp time and completeness of spinal cord revascularization. Clamp time is totally dependent on speed of aortic reconstruction and always should be kept to an absolute minimum. It is our policy to incorporate as many intercostal arteries as is technically feasible during a thoracic aortic reconstruction. Although others have reported methods of localizing critical intercostals contributing to spinal cord blood supply by preoperative angiography or intraoperative techniques, no such efforts yet have been able to prevent paraplegia.[5, 6]

An additional contributor to severity of ischemia is reduction in spinal cord perfusion pressure. Spinal cord perfusion pressure is the difference of the spinal artery pressure minus the cerebrospinal fluid (CSF) pressure. Therefore, perfusion pressure can be augmented by increasing spinal artery pressure or reducing CSF pressure. We maximize flow through collaterals and, hopefully, spinal artery pressure, by maintaining proximal hypertension of 20 to 30 mm Hg higher systolic pressure during clamping as compared with preclamping. We seldom use shunts or bypass to raise the distal aortic pressure because of an increased incidence of complications as well as proven ineffectiveness, as shown by Crawford and others.[7, 8] Spinal fluid pressure increases during aortic clamping, as does the rate of CSF production. To reduce CSF pressure, we use an intrathecal lumbar drain placed after the induction of anesthesia. Initially, 15 mL of CSF are withdrawn; therefore, CSF pressure is maintained at or below 10 mm Hg using a closed collection device. Experimentally, we have documented the protective effect on the spinal cord of CSF drainage in dogs undergoing thoracic aortic clamping.[9, 10] In addition, spinal cord blood flow (as assessed per weight of spinal cord) increases with CSF drainage in dogs.[11] Although others have used CSF drainage without benefit in terms of the incidence of paraplegia,[12] our results are favorable (as discussed later), and we continue to use CSF drainage during all thoracoabdominal aortic procedures.

The central nervous system is very sensitive to ischemic injury because neurons have a higher metabolic demand than do other tissues. The metabolic rate of neural tissue is diminished with reduced temperature. This is well documented by multiple cases of near-drowning in cold water as well as planned hypothermic arrest for some cardiac surgical procedures. In the ischemic spinal cord of rabbits, we demonstrated the protective effect of hypothermia as well as that of barbiturate coma with high-dose thiopental sodium.[13] During thoracoabdominal aortic surgery, we allow the patient's temperature to fall to 32 to 34°C at the time of clamping by keeping the operating room at a comfortable temperature for the surgical team and not using a warming blanket. Fifteen minutes prior to clamping, thiopental sodium (20 mg/kg) is administered intravenously to induce a barbiturate coma. Rewarming efforts with a warming blanket, warming of intravenous fluids, and increased room temperature are started after the revascularization is completed. Furthermore, dextrose administration is avoided, since evidence exists that hyperglycemia potentiates ischemic spinal cord injury.[14]

The role of reperfusion injury in the spinal cord is unclear, but the observation of delayed-onset paraplegia in patients who awaken from anesthesia neurologically normal and then develop a neurologic deficit suggests a role for reperfusion injury. Some investigators have suggested that delayed-onset paraplegia is related to postoperative hemodynamic compromise with reduced spinal cord blood flow. However, we have had two such cases in which no hemodynamic abnormality occurred. Furthermore, in the ischemic spinal cord of rabbits, we and others have observed delayed-onset paraplegia, the risk of which is related to the extent of ischemic injury.[4, 15]

Precise methods of reperfusion injury in the ischemic spinal cord have not been defined. Free radicals, cytotoxic action by leukocytes, edema within the confines of the spinal canal, and spinal vasoconstriction induced by arachidonic acid metabolites all are potential mechanisms by which reperfusion injury could be induced.[16–21] At this time, we provide empiric treatment to minimize reperfusion injury to the spinal cord with mannitol and steroids. Mannitol is a weak free radical scavenger; although more effective free radical scavengers exist, they are not approved yet for general use in humans. Twenty-five grams of mannitol is administered 30 minutes prior to clamping and an additional dose of 12.5 g is given 5 minutes prior to reperfusion. Steroids methylprednisolone [Solumedrol] 30 mg/kg and hydrocortisone 100 mg are administered at the beginning of the procedure for their potential benefit as membrane stabilizers and free radical scavengers. However, it should be emphasized that mannitol and steroids are empiric treatments.

POSTOPERATIVE CARE

Hemodynamic parameters need careful attention postoperatively. The cardiac index is maintained at 2.0 L/min/m^2 or greater with volume support and, when needed, inotropic support. Routine low-dose dopamine is used to augment renal perfusion. Ventilator support for 1 to 3 days is routine, since patients do not awaken from the barbiturate coma until the night of or day following the operation. CSF drainage is continued for 48 to 72 hours postoperatively, with a target CSF pressure of 10 mm Hg. If the CSF pressure rises above 20 mm Hg, 15 cc of CSF is aspirated carefully to reduce the pressure rapidly. Additionally, a careful neurologic assessment is made each hour. Consultation with a neurologist is obtained

TABLE 1.

Risk of Spinal Cord Ischemia in 150 Consecutive Patients Undergoing Operation for Thoracoabdominal Aortic Aneurysm

Number of Patients	Neurologic Deficit				
	Total	Type I	Type II	Type III	Type IV
Overall (%)	8/180 (4.4)	2/35 (5.7)	3/39 (7.7)	2/48 (4.2)	1/58 (1.7)
Preprotocol (%)	6/108 (5.6)	2/22 (9.1)	2/16 (12.5)	2/23 (8.7)	0/47 (0)
Protocol (%)	2/72 (2.8)	0/13 (0)	1/23 (4.3)	0/25 (0)	1/11 (9.1)

if any neurologic dysfunction is noted. Any deterioration in lower-extremity motor function is treated with an additional 15 mL withdrawal of CSF as well as redosing of steroids and mannitol.

CLINICAL RESULTS

Since we instituted this multimodality protocol designed to reduce the risk of spinal cord ischemia in thoracoabdominal aortic surgery, 72 patients have been treated and compared with 108 patients treated prior to development of the protocol. Ninety-seven percent of the patients survived at least long enough to evaluate their neurologic function. Aneurysm types and neurologic injury rates are summarized in Table 1. One case each of acute-onset and delayed-onset paraplegia comprise the neurologic deficits noted in the protocol group. The acute-onset deficit occurred in a patient who suffered intraoperative arrest and in whom intercostal reimplantation was not done in order to expedite the procedure. The delayed-onset deficit was noted 9 days postoperatively in a patient who had become hypoxic and hypotensive earlier in the day.

SUMMARY

No known methods can eliminate entirely the risk of spinal cord injury resulting from thoracoabdominal aortic aneurysm repair. This surgical complication seems to be a result of the severity of ischemia, the metabolic rate of the spinal cord during the period of ischemia, and the extent of reperfusion injury. We have been successful, though, in reducing the incidence of spinal cord injury by using a multimodality protocol during the repair of thoracoabdominal aortic aneurysms.

REFERENCES

1. Hollier LH, Money SR, Naslund TC, et al: The risk of spinal cord dysfunction in 150 consecutive patients undergoing thoracoabdominal aortic replacement. Am J Surg 1992; 164:210–214.
2. Crawford ES, Crawford JL, Safi HJ, et al: Thoracoabdominal aortic aneurysms: Preoperative and intraoperative factors determining immediate and long-term results of operation in 605 patients. J Vasc Surg 1986; 3:389–404.

3. Gray H: *Anatomy of the Human Body.* Philadelphia, Lea & Febiger, 1985, pp 964–976.

4. Moore WM, Hollier LH: The influence of severity of spinal cord ischemia in the etiology of delayed-onset paraplegia. *Ann Surg* 1991; 213:427–432.

5. Kieffer E, Richard R, Chiras J, et al: Preoperative spinal cord arteriography in aneurysmal disease of the descending thoracic and thoracoabdominal aorta: Preliminary results in 45 patients. *Ann Vasc Surg* 1989; 3:34–46.

6. Svensson LG, Patel V, Robinson MF, et al: Influence of preservation or perfusion of intraoperatively identified spinal cord blood supply on spinal motor evoked potentials and paraplegia after aortic surgery. *J Vasc Surg* 1991; 13:355–365.

7. Crawford ES, Mizrahi EM, Hess KR, et al: The impact of distal aortic perfusion and somatosensory evoked potential monitoring on prevention of paraplegia after aortic aneurysm operation. *J Thorac Cardiovasc Surg* 1988; 95:357–367.

8. Livesay JJ, Couley DA, Ventimiglia RA, et al: Surgical experience in descending thoracic aneurysmectomy with and without adjuncts to avoid ischemia. *Ann Thorac Surg* 1985; 39:37–46.

9. Granke K, Hollier LH, Zdrahal P, et al: Longitudinal study of cerebrospinal fluid drainage and polyethylene glycol-conjugated superoxide dismutase in paraplegia associated with thoracic aortic cross-clamping. *J Vasc Surg* 1991; 13:615–621.

10. McCullough JL, Hollier LH, Nugent M: Paraplegia after thoracic aortic occlusion: Influence of cerebrospinal fluid drainage. *J Vasc Surg* 1988; 7:153–160.

11. Bower TC, Murray MJ, Gloviczki P, et al: Effects of thoracic aortic occlusion and cerebrospinal fluid drainage on regional blood flow in dogs: Correlation with neurologic outcome. *J Vasc Surg* 1988; 9:135–144.

12. Crawford ES, Svensson LG, Hess KR, et al: A prospective randomized study of cerebrospinal fluid drainage to prevent paraplegia after high risk surgery on the thoracoabdominal aorta. *J Vasc Surg* 1991; 13:36–46.

13. Naslund TC, Hollier LH, Money SR, et al: Protecting the ischemic spinal cord during aortic clamping: The influence of anesthetics and hypothermia. *Ann Surg* 1992; 215:409–416.

14. Lundy EF, Ball TD, Mandell MA, et al: Dextrose administration increases sensory/motor impairment and paraplegia after infrarenal aortic occlusion in the rabbit. *Surgery* 1987; 102:737–742.

15. Zivin JA, DeGirolami U, Hurwitz EL: Spectrum of neurological deficits in experimental CNS ischemia. A quantitative study. *Arch Neurol* 1982; 39:408–412.

16. Arnfred I, Secher O: Anorexia and barbiturates: Tolerance to anoxia in mice influenced by barbiturates. *Arch Int Pharmacodyn Ther* 1962; 139:67–74.

17. Laschinger JC, Cunningham JN, Cooper MM, et al: Prevention of ischemic spinal cord injury following aortic cross-clamping: Use of corticosteroids. *Ann Thorac Surg* 1984; 38:500–507.

18. Giulian D: Ameboid microglia as effectors of inflammation in the central nervous system. *J Neurosci Res* 1987; 18:155–171.

19. Chen ST, Hsu CY, Hogen EL, et al: Thromboxane, prostacyclin, and leukotrienes in cerebral ischemia. *Neurology* 1986; 36:466–470.

20. Jacobs TP, Shohami E, Baze W, et al: Deteriorating stroke model: Histopathology, edema, and eicosanoid changes following spinal cord ischemia on rabbits. *Stroke* 1982; 18:741–750.

21. Clark WM, Madden KP, Rothlein R, et al: Reduction of central nervous system ischemic injury in rabbits using leukocyte adhesion antibody treatment. *Stroke* 1991; 22:877–883.

PART III

Endovascular Techniques

Endovascular Repair of Abdominal Aortic Aneurysms

JUAN C. PARODI, M.D.

This chapter describes the development of a form of endovascular treatment for abdominal aortic aneurysms (AAAs) and other arterial diseases. My associates and I hope that this information concerning our early animal experimentation and our subsequent series of patients will be of value and, in some way, will be provocative to all clinicians who are responsible for the diagnosis and management of AAAs. We also are pleased to lend our experience to fellow investigators who are engaged in similar research, and we hope that it helps them to avoid a few of the mistakes that we initially made.

The diagnosis of AAA has been established with increasing frequency during the past 2 decades.[1] This observation probably is related to aging of the population, as well as to the extensive use of ultrasonography and computerized tomographic (CT) scanning for screening purposes. Although AAAs occasionally may cause distal embolization to the lower extremities, rupture remains their most common and deadly complication. It has been established that fewer than 30% of all patients who sustain ruptured aneurysms survive this catastrophe, a figure that includes a mortality rate of about 50%, even among those who live long enough to receive urgent surgical intervention.

Elective replacement with a synthetic graft has proved to be the most appropriate method of preventing AAA rupture for nearly 40 years and, at respected medical centers, it has been associated with a postoperative mortality rate of less than 5%, even in high-risk patients.[2] Nevertheless, surgical risk undoubtedly is higher in hospitals at which there is less experience with aortic reconstruction, and nonfatal complications occur with some regularity irrespective of the setting in which the operation is performed. Finally, the decision to recommend elective surgical management is influenced by an infinite number of considerations regarding the likelihood of rupture of untreated AAAs related to their size, as well as to the operative risk in patients who have incidental cardiac, pulmonary, or renal disease.[3] It seems inevitable that every vascular surgeon occasionally will encounter a patient who represents a prohibitive risk for conventional graft replacement, yet alternative forms of treatment (such as axillofemoral bypass in conjunction with induced AAA thrombosis) gen-

Advances in Vascular Surgery, vol. 1.
©1993, Mosby–Year Book, Inc.

erally have been abandoned, despite preliminary reports of their initial success.[4]

In 1976, we began to develop a plan for the endovascular treatment of AAAs that was based upon the fundamental principles of aortic replacement. Our first two prototypes may be described as follows:

1. *A metallic self-expandable mesh with a "zig zag" configuration, covered by a thin fabric graft that was compressed and introduced inside a sheath.* This prototype was employed experimentally in normal canine aortas, but we found that it was difficult to deploy because the elastic properties of the metallic cage were difficult to standardize. If too much radial pressure were applied, damage to the aortic wall eventually could cause its rupture. Conversely, the application of too little pressure permitted subsequent migration of the graft, with leakage of blood between it and the host aorta.

2. *A Silastic bag with a cylindric lumen, fitted within a Dacron graft.* This bag was introduced into simulated AAAs in dogs, and then was distended by the injection of silicone into the bag. Unfortunately, this method was associated with prompt thrombosis of the aorta in all experimental animals.

We eventually abandoned both of these prototypes because of their complications, but we reinitiated our project when balloon-expandable stents became available in 1988. Our current approach is predicated upon the concept that stents may be used in place of sutures to secure the proximal and distal ends of a fabric graft extending the length of the AAA (Fig 1). Balloon-expandable stents appeared to fulfill the necessary re-

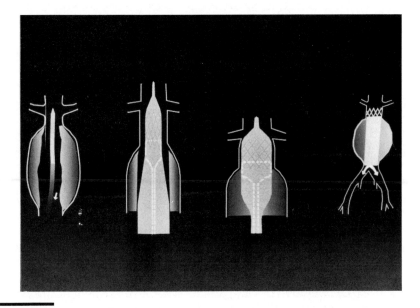

FIGURE 1.

Schematic illustration of the endovascular treatment of abdominal aortic aneurysms.

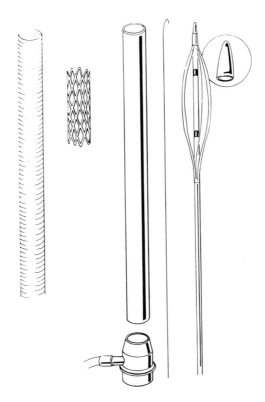

FIGURE 2.

The elements comprising our endovascular device.

quirements for this purpose because their positioning could be calculated precisely, the radial force necessary for their deployment was predictable, and their diameter could be selected to match that of the aorta itself.

The sheath that we employ currently contains the following elements (Fig 2):

1. A single- or double-balloon catheter of appropriate diameter.
2. Mounted over the catheter, a balloon-expandable stent similar to that introduced by Palmaz (Johnson & Johnson, Warren, NJ), but adapted for larger diameters.
3. A knitted, crimped, thin-walled synthetic graft made of Dacron yarn that is comparable in strength to other commercial grafts that already are available.

Once the graft has been introduced transfemorally to the appropriate level of the aorta, either the proximal balloon alone or both the proximal and the distal balloons are inflated in order to fix the graft firmly in place. If our method proves to be safe and durable, it would avoid the complications of general anesthesia, intra-abdominal surgical dissection, blood transfusion, prolonged aortic clamping, and sexual dysfunction related to disturbance of the pelvic autonomic nerves that may be associated with traditional surgical treatment.

LABORATORY EXPERIENCE

In order to determine the feasibility of our proposed method, we performed a number of animal experiments that have been reported elsewhere.[5, 6] In summary, we constructed an artificial AAA by resecting a segment of the infrarenal aorta and replacing it with a fusiform Dacron graft (Fig 3). This model reproduced the important features of human AAAs; that is, endothelium was found to cover the surface of the graft at the "neck" of the experimental aneurysm, and mural thrombus occupied much of the cavity of the dilated segment. Both of these changes were encountered regularly within a month after the experimental AAA had been implanted.

After 4 weeks, these dogs again were placed under general anesthesia and the common femoral artery was exposed. A guidewire was advanced into the suprarenal aorta, and a 14-French sheath containing a Palmaz iliac stent and a Dacron graft mounted on a balloon catheter was placed over the wire. After the sheath had been removed, the endovascular graft was positioned within the experimental AAA and then was secured by deploying either one or two stents (Figs 4 and 5). In one group of dogs, we used only a proximal stent, and in another, we used a second stent at the distal end of the exclusion graft.

We operated on a total of 43 dogs, in most cases to evaluate different

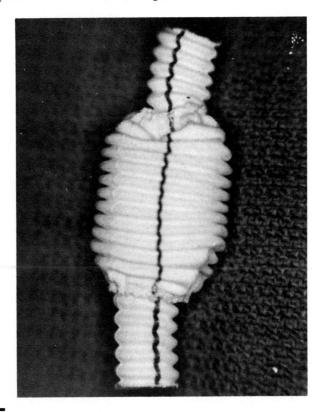

FIGURE 3.

An example of the "artificial aneurysm" constructed using a Dacron conduit in our animal studies.

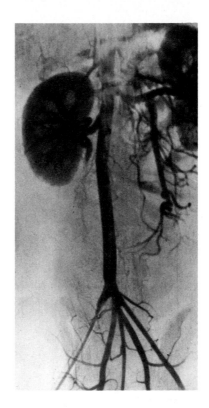

FIGURE 4.
A representative aortogram 4 weeks after the construction of an "artificial aneurysm" in a dog.

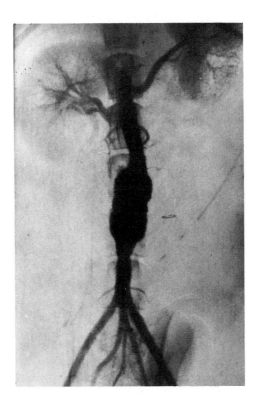

FIGURE 5.
Another aortogram following the implantation of a stented aortic graft through the right femoral artery in the same dog illustrated in Figure 4.

models for experimental aneurysm or to test a variety of balloons and replacement grafts. In our last group of dogs, we performed 6-month evaluations, obtaining color-Doppler ultrasound (duplex) scans in some cases and complete pathologic studies in all animals. Using both optical and electronic microscopy, we found that both ends of the stented grafts were covered by endothelium, and that the shaft of the graft that was in contact with the mural thrombus of the experimental AAA was covered by a fibrin-platelet barrier.

Once we were satisfied that a Dacron graft could be delivered through a catheter and fixed firmly in place by balloon-expandable stents, we obtained the permission of our institutional ethical committee to perform a pilot clinical study with a small group of patients who were informed fully regarding the nature of our work and subsequently were followed very carefully.[7]

CLINICAL EXPERIENCE

DEVICE COMPONENTS

The device used in our clinical work is illustrated in Figure 2. A superstiff guidewire with a diameter of 0.038 in. (Amplatz, Meditech, Boston) facilitates introduction of the device through tortuous iliac arteries, keeps the axis of the device parallel to that of the aorta, and, therefore, tends to prevent disruption of laminated thrombus contained within the AAA. The *balloon-expandable stent* is a cylindric tube with longitudinal slots that adopt a diamond shape when expanded. This design, initially described by Palmaz,[8, 9] permits the stent to expand from a diameter of only 5 mm when collapsed to a diameter of more than 30 mm when expanded. The stent is 3.5 mm in length, and its metallic component represents only 20% of its surface area after deployment.

The *knitted Dacron graft* has a wall thickness of 0.2 mm and is fabricated using strong yarns with tensile and bursting strengths comparable to those of commercially available grafts. The compliance of the shaft of the graft (15%) also is similar to standard, knitted Dacron grafts, but the compliance of the segment overlapping the stent is 45% in order to adapt to its expansion. Between these two segments, a transitional zone of intermediate compliance is interposed in an attempt to avoid abrupt changes in the diameter of the graft that eventually could produce deleterious friction between the stent and the shaft of the graft itself. The diameter and length of each graft is tailored to fit the individual patient, but the grafts we have employed most often are 18 to 20 mm in diameter and 8 to 12 cm in length.

Because of its radiopacity, a thin *gold wire* is knitted to each graft. This permits the radiographic identification of both ends and the sides of the graft in order for us to correct torsion during implantation. The *balloon catheters* have a shaft constructed of polyvinylchloride with a 9-French diameter, and they contain either two or three lumina, depending upon the number of low-profile, nonelastomeric polyethylene balloons affixed to them. If two balloons are used, the caudal one has a cylindric configuration leading into a 30-degree angle in the catheter shaft immediately below it in order to accommodate the typical angle of origin taken by the iliac arteries at the level of the aortic bifurcation. We generally use just two balloon diameters that adapt to an inflated diameter of 18 to 30 mm. Finally, the *Teflon sheath* has a diameter of 21-French and a valve at the proximal end.

PREPROCEDURAL EVALUATION

Our evaluation of patients who may be potential candidates for endovascular treatment is identical to that for those who receive conventional surgical management. A CT scan of the abdominal aorta is performed at 1-cm intervals, usually with additional "cuts" at the proximal and distal extent of the AAA. The CT scan allows us to estimate the distance between the renal arteries and the aortic bifurcation, to calculate the diameter of the aorta at the upper and lower ends of the AAA, and to identify aortic tortuosity or angulation that may influence our approach. In addition, we obtain a biplanar abdominal aortogram in every patient because it provides further detail concerning the visceral branches, the patency of the inferior mesenteric and lumbar arteries, and the course and diameter of the iliac arteries. Angiography is performed using a pigtail catheter with gold calibrations at 2-cm intervals, and a radiopaque ruler also is positioned vertically behind the patient.

The aortogram is interpreted from a perspective focused on the center of the fluoroscopy screen because this precaution minimizes distortion of the image. Most AAAs contain laminated thrombus that typically is distributed in a characteristic fashion. Thrombus usually involves the entire length of the AAA, but ordinarily is most dense in the distal aorta and tends to occlude the ostia of the lumbar and inferior mesenteric arteries at that level. This feature produces an enlarged flow lumen in the proximal AAA, together with a lumen of nearly normal diameter in its distal third. Therefore, unless the angiographic features are supplemented by CT data, the distal neck of the AAA may be considered adequate to secure a stented graft when, in fact, it is not. If we encounter substantial differences in the information concerning length and diameter that we have collected using CT scanning and aortography, we review our data to determine whether an obvious error has been committed. Minor differences are not uncommon, however, and we have found that the CT scan sometimes overestimates the intraluminal diameter of the aorta by a factor of 1 to 4 mm. Once all dimensions have been determined, we are able to design the implantation device to be used in a specific patient.

PROCEDURAL TECHNIQUE

The patient is prepared and draped as though conventional AAA resection were to be performed. Under either local anesthesia or, as we prefer, epidural anesthesia, the common femoral artery is exposed through a standard groin incision ipsilateral to the iliac artery that is straighter and less diseased angiographically. Sodium heparin (5,000 IU) is administered intravenously, and a number 18 Cournand needle is inserted cephalad into the common femoral artery. A soft-tip (0.038-in.) guidewire is advanced through the needle into the distal thoracic aorta, and a 5-French pigtail angiographic catheter is introduced over it. Once the catheter is positioned in the visceral segment of the abdominal aorta, the wire is removed and preprocedural angiography is performed. The pigtail catheter has radiopaque calibrations at 20-mm intervals to obtain measurements from the computer-assisted angiogram, and we again place a radiopaque ruler behind the patient that is parallel to the axis of the aorta. After comparing our measurements to those that were collected previously, the appropriate endoluminal device may be constructed.

The graft overlaps the proximal stent by about two thirds, and is attached to it using braided, synthetic suture material. We now place two sutures on both sides of the graft separated by 180 degrees because we once encountered graft dislodgment when only one suture was used on each side. After mounting the stent(s) over the balloon(s), the graft is folded and the entire assembly is introduced into a 21-French Teflon sheath.

The guidewire is reintroduced, the pigtail catheter is removed, and the original wire is replaced with a super-stiff (Amplatz) wire. Another intravenous dose (5,000 IU) of sodium heparin is administered, and the sheath containing the device is advanced over the new wire to the level of the proximal neck of the AAA (Fig 6). The sheath then is removed, leaving the graft, stent(s), and balloon(s) in the aortic lumen (Fig 7). In order to prevent distal migration during inflation of the proximal balloon, we often initiate an intravenous infusion of nitroglycerin to maintain the mean systemic blood pressure below 100 mm Hg. As soon as the blood pressure is stable at an appropriate level, the proximal balloon is inflated

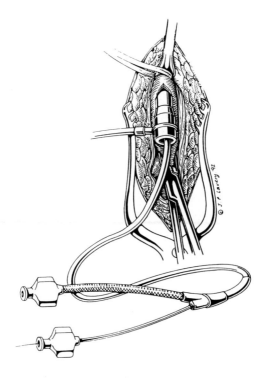

FIGURE 6.

Introduction of the sheath for our clinical device using a femoral arteriotomy.

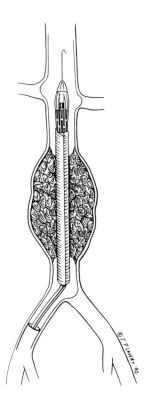

FIGURE 7.
After removal of the sheath, the balloon is positioned for deployment of the stent.

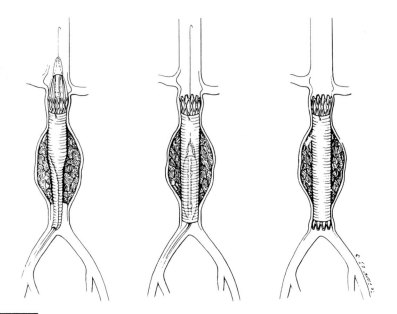

FIGURE 8.
An illustration of the three components of our clinical procedure: proximal stent deployment, distention of the graft, and placement of the distal stent.

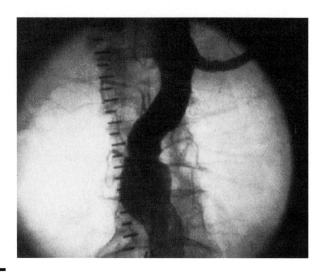

FIGURE 9.

A preprocedural aortogram (patient number 10 in our series).

for 1 minute with whatever volume is necessary to attain the proper diameter for that particular patient. To apply a perfectly cylindric shape to the stent, we occasionally inflate the balloon again at both ends of the stent. None of our patients has experienced discomfort or significant blood pressure changes during balloon inflation. In one of them, we adopted the shape of the stent to an irregular aneurysm neck by making repeated inflations under low pressure along the entire length of the stent.

After the proximal stent has been deployed, we inflate the balloon along the shaft of the graft to distend it under low pressure (Fig 8). Provided all previous measurements were correct, the distal radiopaque calibrations on the graft should be flush to the aortic bifurcation at the con-

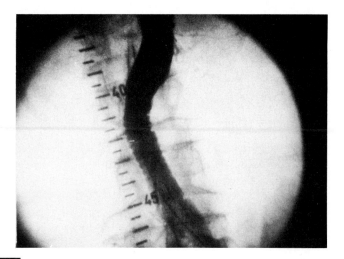

FIGURE 10.

Another aortogram following endovascular grafting in the same patient illustrated in Figure 9.

clusion of the procedure (Figs 9 and 10). A completion aortogram then is obtained. If it demonstrates reflux around the distal end of the graft into the aneurysm sac, a second stent is placed at that level. Special balloons have been designed specifically for this purpose because the distal neck of the AAA usually is short and would not accommodate easily a standard valvuloplasty balloon. These special balloons are cylindric, and their catheters are angulated by 30 degrees near the balloon end of the shaft in order to adapt to the angle at the origin of the common iliac artery. Whenever endovascular grafting is performed in patients who already have sustained previous lower-extremity embolization, we electively use two stents mounted on a double-balloon catheter. After deploying the proximal stent and then deflating its balloon, the distal stent is engaged by inflating the second balloon under slight tension to straighten the graft.

The arteriotomy is closed after flushing the iliac artery to vent any debris that might have been loosened during the procedure. The patient is transferred to an intensive care unit for the next 24 hours, and usually spends 2 additional days on a regular nursing floor before being discharged from the hospital. Antibiotic coverage has been limited to a single dose of cephalothin (Keflin), 1 g intravenously, 30 minutes before the endoluminal procedure.

PATIENT SELECTION

Our clinical experience has been limited to 13 patients, because it was our intention to analyze our results in considerable detail before recommending endoluminal treatment of AAAs on a wide scale. For this reason, we initially selected only those candidates who had serious comorbidities implying a high surgical risk with conventional resection and graft replacement. Although we subsequently accepted a few volunteers who did not represent prohibitive surgical risks, two anatomic criteria must be met under any circumstances:

1. Both the proximal and the distal necks of the AAA must be at least 2 cm in length.
2. At least one of the iliac arteries must be patent and sufficiently straight to access the device. A short segment of iliac stenosis, however, can be corrected by percutaneous transluminal angioplasty (PTA) in conjunction with the endoluminal graft procedure.

We decided not to treat patients who had patent inferior mesenteric or lumbar arteries in our pilot study, but, with these exceptions about half of all the candidates we evaluated met our other anatomic criteria. We presently are investigating the feasibility of endoluminal placement of aortoiliac bifurcation grafts using a modification of our endoluminal approach through both common femoral arteries. If this refinement proves to be successful, we estimate that more than 90% of patients with an AAA eventually could be treated without a traditional operation.

Twelve of our original 13 patients had AAAs, and 1 had a subclavian arteriovenous fistula. There were 12 men and 1 woman in our series. They ranged in age from 62 to 83 years (mean, 71 years), and their follow-up periods extend from 3 to 23 months (mean, 10 months). The results in our first 5 patients have been reported previously.[7]

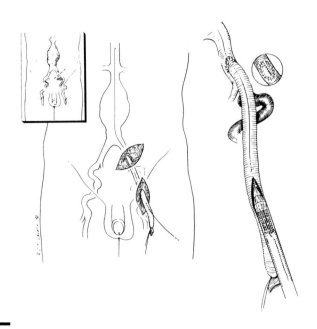

FIGURE 11.

A temporary iliac conduit constructed using a 10-mm Dacron graft to facilitate the introduction of a 21-French sheath.

Ten of the 13 patients were considered to be high-risk candidates for standard AAA resection and refused conventional operations, and the remaining 3 patients volunteered to be included in our protocol. Risk factors included recent myocardial infarction, hemorrhagic brain infarction, and pulmonary edema (each in 1 patient); another patient had chronic renal failure. Six patients had chronic pulmonary insufficiency, and another 6 had severe coronary artery disease. All of the patients and their close relatives were informed fully concerning our method and its perceived risks, and all gave written consent.

The procedures were performed in our cardiac laboratory under ei-

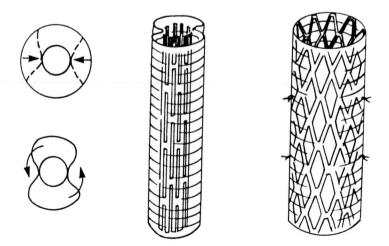

FIGURE 12.

An endovascular stent covered by a Dacron graft.

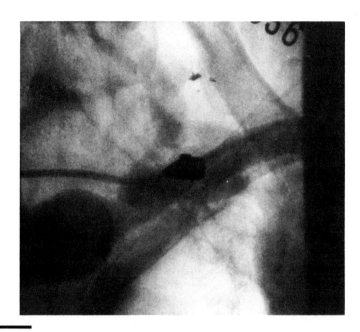

FIGURE 13.
A preprocedural angiogram demonstrating a subclavian arteriovenous fistula caused by a gunshot wound.

ther epidural (12 patients) or local anesthesia. Three of these procedures were supplemented by PTA of the iliac artery and another two by segmental graft replacement of common femoral aneurysms. Our initial attempt to introduce the sheath failed in 2 patients, but, in each case, the contralateral iliac artery was employed successfully. Transfemoral access

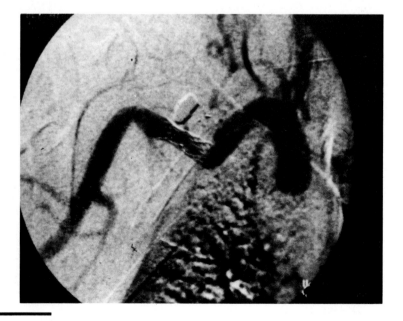

FIGURE 14.
Another angiogram following endovascular grafting in the same patient illustrated in Figure 13.

from either side was impossible in only 1 patient. In this case, we made a short, extraperitoneal incision to perform an anastomosis between the common iliac artery and a straight Dacron graft that provided a conduit for the sheath (Fig 11). After the stented aortic graft had been implanted, the iliac graft was removed, with the exception of a short segment that simply was oversewn near its iliac anastomosis.

One interesting 62-year-old patient was referred for treatment with the mistaken diagnosis of a subclavian aneurysm. In fact, he had sustained a gunshot wound 2 years earlier and subsequently had developed an arteriovenous fistula manifest by a pulsatile subclavian mass, a prominent subcutaneous venous pattern, and hyperdynamic cardiomegaly. At his request, we inserted our device through a sheath in the ipsilateral axillary artery in order to implant a short endoluminal Dacron graft using a 10-mm balloon deployed directly at the site of the fistula itself (Fig 12). All obvious manifestations of the previous fistula (thrill, bruit, and tachycardia) resolved as soon as the graft was inserted, and an immediate arteriogram confirmed the closure of the fistula. Another arteriogram obtained 1 month later demonstrated a patent subclavian artery without any apparent abnormalities (Figs 13 and 14).

COMPLICATIONS

There were no deaths related to our procedures, and all of our patients have remained alive throughout our current follow-up period.

We have encountered six nonfatal complications in 5 of our 13 patients:

1. *Inguinal hematoma.* This complication occurred only once, probably

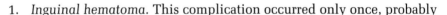

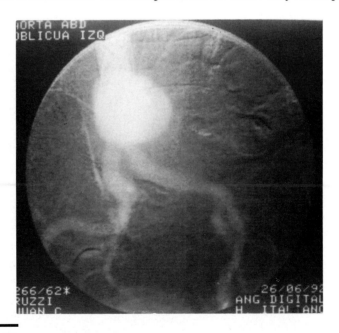

FIGURE 15.

An aortogram demonstrating dilation of the distal abdominal aorta 18 months after endovascular implantation of a Dacron graft having inadequate length.

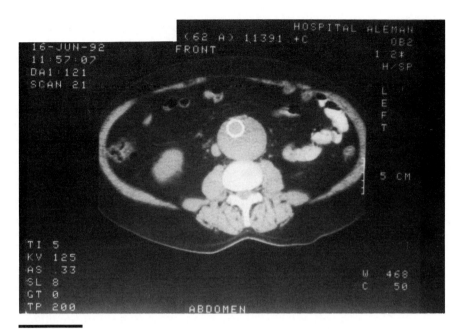

FIGURE 16.

A computed tomographic scan after deployment of a distal stent that engaged only the mural thrombus in the same patient illustrated in Figure 15.

was related to the fact that we did not reverse systemic heparinization at the conclusion of the first procedure in our series, and has not recurred since we have begun routine administration of postprocedural protamine sulfate.

2. *Malpositioning of the proximal stent.* This complication occurred in the second patient in our series and represented a technical error on the part of the interventionalist. This oversight could be corrected only by standard AAA resection and graft replacement, and it was during this operation that we recognized that surgical removal of an implanted stent is quite difficult (see later). Nevertheless, this particular patient had an uneventful postoperative course.

3. *Leakage through the proximal stent.* As indicated earlier, we initially secured our graft to its stent with only two sutures positioned 180 degrees apart. In such a case, one of the sutures loosened and permitted the graft to migrate distally on that side. After identifying this problem during the procedure, we successfully deployed another stented Dacron graft within the lumen of the displaced graft. This patient had no further complications.

4. *Miscalculation of graft length.* In another patient, the first graft we implanted was too short to reach the distal neck of the AAA. Once again, we deployed a second stented graft of appropriate length within the lumen of the original graft in order to solve this problem.

5. *Distal graft reflux.* We identified reflux of blood into the aneurysm sac at the distal end of the implanted graft in the fourth patient in our series, but we chose to terminate the procedure with the expectation that this finding might resolve spontaneously. This proved to

be an error in judgment, because it became necessary to deploy a second stent at the distal end of the graft when reflux still was found to be present 1 month later. Unfortunately, we failed to appreciate that this additional stent was in contact only with laminated mural thrombus, rather than with the true aortic wall. As a result, this patient eventually developed yet another complication. About 18 months later, the patient was found to have further dilation of the distal aorta (Figs 15 and 16). During a standard corrective operation, we found that the proximal end of the endovascular graft was secured firmly to the upper neck of the AAA. Accordingly, we merely replaced its distal end with a new Dacron graft, using a conventional sutured anastomosis at the level of the aortic bifurcation. This patient also recovered uneventfully.

LATE RESULTS

Our follow-up protocol requires a clinical examination, standard laboratory studies, and both color-duplex and CT scans of the implanted grafts every 6 months. Subsequent aortography has been performed in only 5 of our 13 patients (4 of these on a routine basis, and the other in the patient who developed distal aortic dilation), but, in the future, we plan to obtain at least one late angiographic study for every patient in our series.

Conceding the fact that two additional operations were necessary to correct early or late complications of our endovascular method, all of our patients are alive and appear to have no other postprocedural problems during follow-up periods ranging from 3 to 23 months (mean, 10 months). On the basis of our present experience, color-duplex scanning seems to be just as accurate as CT scanning for long-term surveillance.

TECHNICAL CONSIDERATIONS

ARTERIAL ACCESS

Occlusion, stenosis, or tortuosity of the iliac arteries obviously provides an obstacle to endovascular management of AAAs, and it already has been necessary for us to perform iliac PTA to correct stenotic lesions prior to the insertion of our device in three patients. In our limited experience, tortuosity of the iliac arteries is related directly to AAA size in the sense that larger AAAs tend to cause more elongation and redundancy of both the aorta and its bifurcation vessels. We have developed a sequential approach to overcome the access problems related to this particular situation:

1. *Use of an Amplatz super-stiff guidewire.* Mild iliac tortuosity often responds to this simple technique.
2. *Circumferential dissection of the common femoral and external iliac arteries.* Once all minor branches of the common femoral artery and the external iliac artery near the inguinal ligament have been ligated and divided, gentle traction downward may straighten the proximal segment of the external iliac artery sufficiently to permit insertion of our device (Fig 17).
3. *Construction of a temporary iliac conduit.* In one of our patients, it

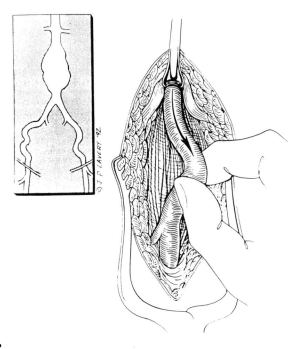

FIGURE 17.

Traction upon the iliac artery to straighten its tortuosity.

was necessary to perform an end-to-side anastomosis of a 10-mm, collagen-coated Dacron graft to the common iliac artery through a short, extraperitoneal incision. This graft then was passed into the groin through an anatomic tunnel anterior to the native arteries before it was used to insert the stented aortic graft. After the procedure had been completed, the temporary conduit was divided, oversewn near its iliac anastomosis, and removed.

Most of the characteristics of the Palmaz stent make it especially adaptable to the endovascular treatment of AAAs. It provides an appropriate radial force to anchor its overlapping graft reliably at the proximal neck, and it has an established record of success in conjunction with PTA of the iliac arteries. Nevertheless, its rigidity sometimes makes it difficult to negotiate a Palmaz stent into the aorta through tortuous iliac arteries, a problem that is particularly evident with longer stents. Because only short stents are necessary to "seal" the distal anastomosis of an endovascular graft, flexibility is an important consideration, principally with respect to the longer (3.5-cm) stents that we have used to secure our grafts firmly at the proximal neck of the AAA.

Several refinements of current stents may be necessary. It may be feasible to construct articulated stents that would conform to tortuosity within the iliac system. Alternatively, it also may be possible to construct long, highly flexible stents covered with Dacron fabric that could be used for endovascular replacement of the entire infrarenal segment of the aorta in addition to the ipsilateral common iliac artery. In this case, distal migration of the endovascular graft would be prevented both by the anchoring mechanism at the proximal neck and by a reduction in the diameter of the fabric-coated stent in the iliac artery beyond the aortic bifurcation.

DISTAL GRAFT DEPLOYMENT

It is imperative that reflux of blood flow into the aneurysm sac be prevented by proper alignment of the endovascular graft with a normal segment of aorta near its bifurcation. In our experience, this complication does not occur, provided that a distal neck of the AAA is present and a graft of adequate diameter has been tailored to a length that is appropriate to reach it. If these criteria are not satisfied, however, reflux into the sac is common.

Several factors influence the functional length of an implanted endovascular graft. Clearly, an allowance must be made for *tortuosity of the aorta* while tailoring the graft. Furthermore, *crimping of the graft* imparts an element of "memory" to its fabric, resulting in slight loss of length once the graft has been released from tension inside the catheter sheath. Finally, *radial expansion of the graft* occurs after deployment and also compromises its length. Unless all these features are taken into account, the distal end of the graft may be in contact only with mural thrombus rather than with the aortic wall, a situation that theoretically would offer no protection against either continued expansion or rupture of the AAA.

Even if the length of the endovascular graft has been calculated precisely, the anatomy of the AAA itself has important implications regarding whether high-pressure reflux of blood will occur into the aneurysm sac. In general, large aneurysms are less likely than are small aneurysms to have an adequate distal neck, irrespective of their angiographic appearance. Therefore, assumptions in this regard should be made principally on the basis of objective information generated by ultrasonography, CT scanning, or magnetic resonance imaging. In the future, it may be possible to implant bifurcated endovascular grafts through a bifemoral approach, and we also have begun to investigate the use of metallic support (tantalum or gold) for Dacron grafts that would provide sufficient malleability to secure a tubular graft to even a short segment of normal, distal aorta.

At the present time, however, distal stenting usually is necessary in the presence of a short neck near the level of the aortic bifurcation, and we also prefer its use in patients who previously have sustained lower-extremity embolization of mural thrombus. Distal stenting may be done either with a prefabricated double-balloon catheter that is angulated at 30 degrees to accommodate to the origin of the common iliac artery, or with a second, single-balloon catheter that is capable of positioning a short, distal stent near the aortic bifurcation. If a second catheter is used, it must be introduced carefully into the distal graft so as not to displace the graft upward into the aneurysm sac.

PATENT BRANCH VESSELS

We have assumed thus far that the endovascular treatment of AAAs is contraindicated in the presence of patent major branches (e.g., the inferior mesenteric artery) demonstrated by angiography, because retrograde flow from such branches could continue to cause expansion of the excluded aneurysm sac. This assumption is based in part upon our anecdotal experience with two popliteal aneurysms in other patients for which we performed conventional bypass procedures in conjunction with proximal and distal ligation of the popliteal artery, only to observe further expansion of the excluded aneurysms caused by patent geniculate vessels.

Although it is conceivable that spontaneous thrombosis would occur in the inferior mesenteric artery or other, similar branches once endovascular grafting of an AAA had been performed, the fact that such thrombosis is not always observed in the popliteal segment has encouraged us to be cautious in our selection of patients. To clarify this issue, we are in the process of studying the behavior of patent branches following endovascular aortic grafting in a canine model.

SECONDARY ENDOVASCULAR PROCEDURES

Only 1 of our 13 patients has required formal surgical intervention to correct a technical problem directly involving the proximal endovascular stent, but our experience with this case suggests that the presence of a stent can make a standard remedial operation exceedingly difficult. Because it was impossible in this particular patient to apply a vascular clamp to the segment of the aorta that contained the stent, it was necessary to obtain proximal arterial control with an endoluminal balloon inserted through the stented graft. Furthermore, we almost were unable to remove the stent in order to construct a conventional sutured anastomosis for a replacement graft below the renal arteries, despite the fact that this operation was performed as soon as we recognized the complication involving the previous stented graft. If a longer period had elapsed before surgical treatment had been undertaken, we might have been faced with two unfavorable alternatives: to risk irreparable damage to the proximal neck of the AAA by forcefully removing the stent, or to risk eventual disruption of the proximal suture line by constructing it through the metallic mesh of the retained stent.

For all these reasons, we have concluded that technical problems related to endovascular grafting probably should be corrected by *secondary endovascular procedures* whenever possible. The following represent a few indications for such an approach:

1. *Proximal graft migration.* As indicated previously, we encountered asymmetric migration of one side of a graft that we had secured to the proximal stent with a total of only two sutures. We promptly corrected this complication by deploying a second stented graft inside the one that had become displaced, and we have had no further complications of this kind since we began to employ four sutures (two on each side) between the graft and its underlying stent.

2. *Stent deformities.* In our preliminary animal experiments, we observed occasional, elliptic deformities of the proximal stent after 6 months of implantation in dogs that might have been related to external compression. We have not encountered similar findings in our clinical series yet, but, if they were to occur, blood flow under systemic pressure could reenter the excluded aneurysm sac and cause

its further expansion. Under these circumstances, we would attempt to salvage the situation by percutaneous balloon dilatation of the proximal stent to restore its original oval configuration.

3. *Inadequate graft length.* In another of our patients, the length of the initial stented graft was inadequate to reach the distal aortic bifurcation. Once again, it was possible to correct this miscalculation by deploying a second endovascular graft of appropriate length within the lumen of the first one.

MISCELLANEOUS COMPLICATIONS

There are several theoretic complications of endovascular treatment for AAAs with which we have had no experience in our pilot clinical series:

1. *Balloon rupture.* There seem to be two nonsurgical strategies to correct this potential complication. First, provided the proximal stent has not been partially expanded, the entire device could be returned to its sheath and removed. Second, if the stent already has been distended to a diameter that prevents its withdrawal into the sheath, the procedure could be completed by advancing a new, low-profile balloon on the guidewire to replace the ruptured balloon.

2. *Distal embolization.* We thus far have avoided this potential complication by using an Amplatz super-stiff guidewire in order to prevent disruption of mural thrombus by keeping the sheath containing our stented grafts parallel to the axis of the AAA. If emboli were to occur into the iliofemoral arterial segment on the same side through which our device had been introduced, they could not disperse distally beyond our arteriotomy and could be removed before its closure using a conventional embolectomy catheter. Contralateral embolization, however, obviously would represent a serious problem requiring immediate recognition, appropriate angiographic studies, and prompt surgical treatment for its correction. Because of the possibility of such an event, the endovascular management of AAAs should be conducted in a surgical environment that contains both the appropriate radiologic equipment and an available operating suite.

3. *Graft dilation or rupture.* Fabric "fatigue" allows an element of long-term dilation to occur in virtually every knitted Dacron graft. Although we have not detected this phenomenon yet in our clinical series, it conceivably also could occur in our stented graft. If substantial dilation were to develop under surveillance, our previous experience with secondary endovascular procedures seems to indicate that a dilated graft could be replaced by deploying a new stented graft inside the lumen of the old one.

THE FUTURE OF ENDOVASCULAR GRAFTING

We generally have confined the clinical applications of our device to patients who are poor candidates for traditional surgical treatment of their AAAs. Nevertheless, if the late results of stented grafts prove to be successful, the future indications for endovascular management undoubtedly will be extended to include many other patients because of its cost-effectiveness and low morbidity. In an attempt to place the role of stented grafts into proper perspective, we plan to initiate a prospectively randomized study of endovascular treatment vs. noninterventional observation in a series of patients with small AAAs. Since standard resection and graft replacement of such aneurysms is the subject of considerable debate, we may find that endovascular treatment represents an efficient compromise from the standpoints of both patient safety and health care expenditures.

We anticipate that substantial technical refinements in endovascular grafting will occur within the foreseeable future. Three-dimensional images provided by magnetic resonance angiography and intraluminal ultrasonography may make it possible to obtain highly accurate preprocedural measurements from which the length of graft that should be employed in individual patients can be calculated. Furthermore, although the thickness of synthetic grafts historically has not been an important consideration, the potential usefulness of endovascular treatment for AAAs should stimulate industrial research to develop a strong, crimped Dacron fabric that is sufficiently *thin* for implantation through a catheter sheath. Ideally, it also may be feasible to manufacture a malleable graft constructed of both Dacron and metallic yarn (perhaps gold or tantalum) that would adapt precisely to the inner surface of the aortic bifurcation and, therefore, supplant the need for a distal stent.

It also will be necessary to develop flexible balloon-expandable stents or articulated rigid stents in order to overcome the constraints that are associated with the insertion of endovascular grafts in patients who have tortuous iliac arteries. Finally, some solution is necessary for patients who have either tandem iliac aneurysms, or sufficient dilation or redundancy of the aneurysm sac at the distal end of large AAAs that endovascular deployment of a tubular graft presently is impossible. We are pursuing the development of stented bifurcation grafts and a technique for their implantation through a bilateral femoral approach in an effort to extend the potential benefit of endovascular management to a larger number of patients with AAAs. The presence of stented grafts within medium-sized iliac arteries, however, eventually may provoke hyperplastic stenosis for which still another solution will be necessary.

Other possible applications of the graft-stent combination (some of which we already have explored) include the treatment of arteriovenous fistulas and arterial dissections or injuries, and the development of an "internal bypass" for vessels previously treated by PTA. Provided our initial experience with the management of an arteriovenous fistula was representative, endovascular grafting may become the preferred approach for such lesions because of its simplicity and relative safety, and because it avoids the blood loss that often is associated with difficult dissection during their surgical repair. It eventually also may be possible to repair suprarenal aortic aneurysms using stented grafts once suitable techniques have been established for the management of patent visceral branches. This particular application of endovascular treatment would require further refinements in preprocedural measurements and stent technology, but such developments theoretically are possible and probably will occur in the near future.

REFERENCES

1. Melton LJ, Bickerstaff LK, Hollier LH, et al: Changing incidence of abdominal aortic aneurysms: A population-based study. *Am J Epidemiol* 1984; 120:379–386.
2. Brown OW, Hollier LH, Paiarolero PC, et al: Abdominal aortic aneurysm and coronary artery disease: A reassessment. *Arch Surg* 1981; 116:1484–1488.
3. McCombs RP, Roberts B: Acute renal failure after resection of abdominal aortic aneurysm. *Surg Gynecol Obstet* 1979; 148:175–179.
4. Karmody AL, Leather RP, Goldman M, et al: The current position of non-resection treatment for abdominal aortic aneurysms. *Surgery* 1983; 94:591–597.
5. Parodi JC, Palmaz JC, Barone HD: Tratmiento endoluminal de los aneurismas de aorta abdominal. Presented at II Convencion de Cirujanos Vasculares de Habla Hispana, Buenos Aires, Argentina, October 1990.
6. Parodi JC, Palmaz JC, Barone HD: Transluminal aneurysm bypass: Experimental observations and preliminary clinical experiences. Presented at International Congress IV. Endovascular Therapy in Vascular Disease, Scottsdale, Arizona, February 1991.
7. Parodi JC, Palmaz JC, Barone HD: Transfemoral intraluminal graft implantation for abdominal aortic aneurysms. *Ann Vasc Surg* 1991; 5:491–499.
8. Palmaz JC, Richter GM, Noeldge G, et al: Intraluminal stents in atherosclerotic iliac artery stenosis: Preliminary report of multicenter study. *Radiology* 1988; 168:727–731.
9. Rees CR, Palmaz JC, Garcia O, et al: Angioplasty and stenting of completely occluded iliac arteries. *Radiology* 1989; 172:953–959.

Intravascular Stents

JULIO C. PALMAZ, M.D.

FRANK J. RIVERA, M.D.

CARLOS ENCARNACION, M.D.

Intravascular stents are used in general as a mechanical means to solve the most common shortcomings of percutaneous balloon angioplasty: elastic recoil and intimal dissection. The fact that intravascular stents become embedded in the arterial wall by tissue growth weeks to months after placement first was reported by Dotter in 1969. This favorable outcome occurs consistently with any stent design, provided it has a reasonably low metal surface and does not obstruct flow. Endothelium grows over the fibrin-coated metal surface until a continuous endothelial layer covers the stent surface, in weeks to months. Endothelium renders the thrombogenic metal surface protected from thrombus deposition, which is likely to form with slow or turbulent flow. This is an important advantage of intravascular stents over other prosthetic conduits, which never endothelialize in patients, except for a few millimeters beyond the anastomoses. However, early stent failure may occur in situations of slow or turbulent flow, which compounds the thrombogenicity of the stent material. This is a definite risk before endothelialization is complete. The following is an overview of the basic issues of intravascular stenting and a brief review of its clinical application in the noncoronary circulation.

Intravascular stents are named after a British dentist, Charles R. Stent, who died at the turn of the century and who had otherwise nothing to do with these devices. Stent's contribution was the invention of a dental impression material that later was used to support healing skin grafts. The word "stent" eventually was applied to all devices used for the support of living tissues during the healing phase, including internal structures.

The original idea of placing an intravascular stent through a catheter guided under fluoroscopy must be attributed to Charles T. Dotter, who reported the technique in 1969.[1] Twelve years later, a second report, also by Dotter, marked the beginning of a series of publications that extended to the present.

Dotter's original stent was a tightly wound coil spring of stainless steel wire mounted coaxially over a guidewire and it was placed with the aid of a pusher/catheter. Dotter was the first to demonstrate that intravascular stents can be incorporated into the arterial wall and remain patent for a long time. In 1983, Dotter and colleagues introduced the concept of a thermoplastic stent consisting of a small-diameter coil made of the alloy nitinol, which has the ability to change shape when exposed to

Advances in Vascular Surgery, vol. 1.
©1993, Mosby–Year Book, Inc.

increased temperature. The same year, Craag and associates reported a similar device. In 1984, a West German surgeon, Dirk Maass, and his colleagues reported their experimental results with spring-loaded stainless steel coils that increase their diameter by unwinding after release. In 1985, Wright and coworkers described an elastic stent consisting of a tempered stainless steel wire bent into a zigzag tubular configuration (Fig 1). The same year, Palmaz and associates introduced the balloon-expandable stent, a tubular meshwork of annealed stainless steel that is deployed by inflation of a coaxial balloon. In 1987, a spring-loaded meshwork stent was introduced by Sigwart and colleagues. The deployment of this device is accomplished by withdrawing a rolling membrane, allowing the stent to increase its diameter. During the same year, a balloon-expandable tantalum-woven stent was introduced by Strecker and coworkers. Also in that same year, Rabkin and colleagues from the National Academy of Science in Moscow reported their large clinical experience with a nitinol coil stent. In 1988, Robinson and associates proposed a new balloon-expandable stent consisting of interdigitating wire loops similar to a book binding.

More recently, reports of a number of other stents have been published. Among them, the Wiktor-Medtronic (San Diego) balloon-expandable tantulum stent has received preliminary application in patients. A number of nonmetallic stents have been reported, such as the Slepian intravascular paving device and the Mayo Clinic biodegradable stent. An additional concept in intravascular stent placement was introduced with the Gaspardt temporary stent (Lille, France), the stent that can be relocated (Tokorazawa, Japan), and the removable stent (Univer-

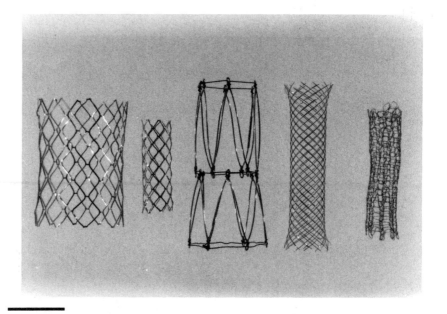

FIGURE 1.

Photographs of the stents most commonly used in the peripheral circulation. From left to right: large and medium-sized Palmaz stents, Gianturco 'Z' stent, Medinvent stent, and Strecker stent.

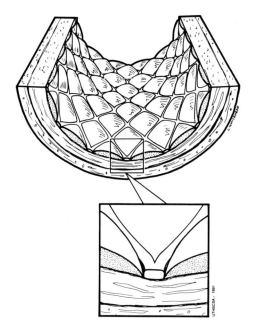

FIGURE 2.

Schematic representation of a well-embedded stent. Insert depicts the trough or depression produced by a strut.

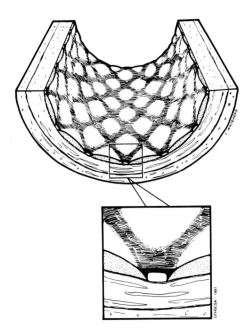

FIGURE 3.

Thrombus deposition in the troughs or depressions of embedded stent.

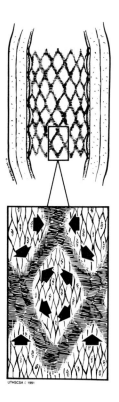

FIGURE 4.

Endothelial cells remaining after stent placement spread in a multicentric fashion.

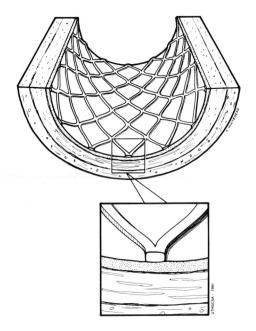

FIGURE 5.

Stent not embedded in the arterial wall. Insert depicts a strut protruding into the vessel lumen.

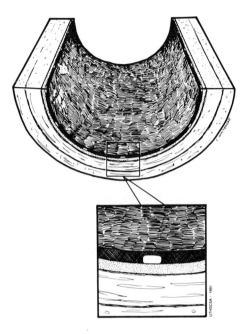

FIGURE 6.

Thrombus covers the entire stented surface in a continuous fashion.

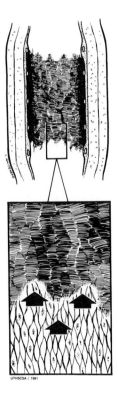

FIGURE 7.

Endothelialization proceeds from the ends of the stented surface.

sity of Pennsylvania). Some of the recently reported stents are in the initial stages of feasibility studies, and others have started to undergo clinical trials.

MECHANICAL CONSIDERATIONS

When stents are applied against the arterial wall, it is most important that the metal members or struts are embedded in the wall away from the circumference of the lumen (Fig 2). The troughs or linear depressions produced are filled rapidly with the thrombus that covers the metal surface. The edges of the thrombus feather toward the tissue mounds protruding between the troughs (Fig 3). These mounds, depending on the degree of blockage and instrumentation prior to stent placement, may retain endothelial cells, allowing reendothelialization by multicentric growth (Fig 4). To embed the stent struts, the balloon diameter chosen for the final expansion of the stent must be 10% to 15% larger than the matched diameter of the vessel adjacent to the target point. If the stent is deployed without this slight overexpansion, the struts will not become embedded (Fig 5) and thrombus will deposit in a continuous layer throughout the surface containing the stent (Fig 6). This entails loss of the endothelium on the treated surface. Reendothelialization, therefore, must proceed from the ends of the deendothelialized area or side branch ostia and is, by ne-

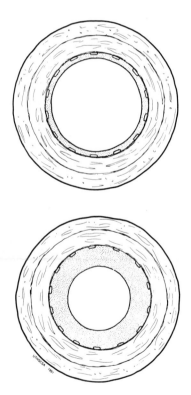

FIGURE 8.

Rapid reendothelialization results in thinner intimal layer (*top*) as compared to slow reendothelialization, thicker intima, and reduced lumen (*bottom*).

cessity, much slower (Fig 7). Slower reendothelialization results in increased thrombus deposition, proliferation of muscle cells, and decreased luminal diameter (Fig 8).

HEMODYNAMIC CONSIDERATIONS

After stent placement, the wall with the stent is rendered rigid by the stent and the ensuing fibromuscular encasement. This loss of radial compliance defeats the ability of musculoelastic vessels to adapt to variable flow and pressure situations. In the case of atherosclerotic vessels, this function already is altered; therefore, stents are not supposed to alter local hemodynamics significantly. In addition to the variable thrombogenic situations outlined in the previous section, freshly implanted stents are subject to increased thrombus deposition in slow-flow situations. This phenomenon was illustrated by Sauvage,[2] who pointed out that thrombus formation over a prosthetic surface is self-limited if flow velocity is maintained above a certain thrombogenic threshold.

Whenever flow drops below this level, thrombus deposits, reducing the lumen. This causes the flow velocity to increase. If the increased flow is above the thrombogenic threshold, thrombus deposition stops. Otherwise, it progresses to the point of complete occlusion. This illustrates the need to attain brisk flow in a newly placed stent by supporting outflow vessel patency and avoiding arterial spasm.

As with prosthetic tubes, the patency rates of stents are likely to be dependent on their diameter, but a somewhat different principle applies to stents in regard to diameter-dependent thrombosis. At the University of Texas, San Antonio, we studied the degree of thrombus deposition over 1.5 to 6.0-mm—diameter canine arteries with stents using the same stent device expanded to match the vessel lumen.[3] Morphometric and radioisotope studies indicated that the amount of thrombus formed was independent of the diameter. We concluded that thrombus material deposited predominantly over the metal surface. Since this surface was identical among stents of variable diameter, the same amount of thrombus material was spread over a larger surface in larger-diameter stents. According to a simple diameter-volume relationship, this amount of thrombus material was relatively occlusive in small stents, although it caused no significant diameter reduction in larger stents.

ANTICOAGULATION AND STENT THROMBOGENICITY

All metals or alloys used in the stents currently under evaluation have electropositive surface in an ionic medium. Although oxides form on the metal surface, the positive surface potential is one of the reasons for electrostatic attraction of negatively charged blood cells and serum proteins. Other factors contributing to stent thrombogenicity are free surface energy and surface texture.[4]

The thrombogenicity of stents decreases a few hours after placement, after the metal surface is covered by thrombus material, which itself constitutes a less thrombogenic surface. This was suggested by time-activity curves of In-111/platelet studies showing peak activity at 60 minutes, followed by a decrease.[5] Further decrease occurs hours to days later as a result of replacement of the amorphous red thrombus material by fibrin thrombus material composed of strands oriented in the direction of flow.[6]

Thrombus formation may be altered drastically with use of anticoagulants and inhibitors of platelet activity. This was shown experimentally in our laboratory. We studied thrombus formation with In-111–labeled platelets in canine femoral stents under different antithrombotic drug regimens as compared with nontreated animals.[3] The amount of radioactivity in the area with a stent was decreased significantly with use of intravenous heparin as compared with that in nontreated animals. Activity was reduced by the addition of aspirin and dipyridamole, but it was depressed maximally by combinations of aspirin and dipyridamole, and intravenous heparin and dextran.

This regimen is recommended to prevent acute stent thrombotic occlusion in situations of slow flow or in stents with diameters smaller than 5 mm, such as those used in the coronary arteries.

RELATIONSHIP BETWEEN SLOW FLOW AND INTIMAL HYPERPLASIA

Although some investigators argue that excessive intimal hyperplasia leading to stent stenosis may be the result of local inflammatory reaction to the metal and/or stimulated smooth muscle cell proliferation, we have found convincing evidence that the thickness of the thrombus over the surface of a stent determines the ultimate thickness of fibromuscular tissue. In a collaborative project between the universities of Freiburg and San Antonio, it was demonstrated experimentally—by means of histologic studies at timely intervals—that a slow flow–induced subocclusive thrombus evolves into fibromuscular tissue. When slow-flow arteries containing a stent are examined 6 months after stent placement, the thick tissue layer covering the stent is indistinguishable from the so-called intimal hyperplasia.[5] If this theory is assumed to be correct, an argument can be made in favor of prolonged anticoagulation with coumarin in situations of slow flow. Evidence against this theory may be seen in well-documented cases of late stent restenosis. However, a late thrombotic cause still may be explained on the basis of discontinuation of coumarin therapy or persistence of absent or dysfunctional endothelium on the segment with a stent. As with other aspects of intravascular stent placement, good judgment and experience may help to identify those patients needing prolonged anticoagulation and frequent controls.

COATED STENTS

A few authors have proposed the application of coats of materials with different properties to metal stents. On the basis of reported work, coats can be classified into passive, active, and biologic. Passive coatings include materials of decreased thrombogenicity such as urethanes and pyrolytic carbon. Active coatings involve materials that are attached chemically to anticoagulants, such as heparin, or have a meshwork structure that may incorporate active substances, including anticoagulants and chemotherapeutic agents. An in vitro biologic coating in the form of seeded endothelial cells on metal stents was reported by Dichek and colleagues.[7] These cells also were genetically engineered to produce tissue plasminogen activator. Although coating appears to be a promising new way to solve an old problem, difficulties are likely to arise. Coatings may present problems with peeling or sloughing. Fluid seepage under the coat also may increase the likelihood of metal corrosion. In the case of endothelial cell coating, the logistic problems related to live cell seeding may be insurmountable.

Assuming that a safe and effective antithrombogenic coating could be developed, questions about its role remain. Endothelium aggressively covers fibrin-coated metal surfaces, but does not grow on polymeric surfaces such as Dacron, Teflon, or Silastic (Dow Corning, Midland, Michigan). By coating stents, we may decrease thrombus formation, but this may result in delayed or incomplete endothelialization, defeating the purpose of its use. Long-term experimental studies must be completed before human application of coated stents is contemplated.

A continuous envelope of Silastic has been applied to balloon-expandable stents to render them impervious to flow through its mesh. This "enveloped" stent was designed for the occlusion of arteriovenous fistulas or saccular aneurysms. However, the polymer surface did not endothelialize, and tissue grew at the ends of the stent lumen when placed in rabbit aortas. As endothelium failed to grow on the plastic surface, layers of thrombus were formed at the transition areas between vessel and the prosthetic surface. The thrombus was replaced progressively but incompletely by fibromuscular tissue in a continuous process perpetuated by the endothelial cell slough.

INTRALUMINAL BYPASS

Stents may be used as friction seals to replace suture in order to affix bypass conduits. This stent-graft combination can be mounted over a coaxial balloon and may be deployed intraluminally to exclude aortic aneurysms. This device was tried in experimentally created abdominal aortic aneurysms in dogs.[8] Six weeks after replacement of a segment of abdominal aorta by a fusiform Dacron conduit to mimic an abdominal aortic aneurysm, an 8-mm segment of crimped, thin-walled graft was introduced through a 12-French Teflon sheath inserted by femoral arteriotomy. Balloon-expandable 3 × 30-mm stents were affixed to the graft ends by two diametrically opposed sutures. The stent-graft assembly was mounted coaxially over a 10-mm × 12-cm balloon angioplasty catheter. After positioning the assembly at the level of the aneurysm, a single balloon inflated expanded the stents and graft, simultaneously excluding the aneurysm. Pathologic examination of the specimens 6 months after placement of the device showed consistent shrinkage of the Dacron experimental aneurysm due to fibrous infiltration. This caused variable degrees of kinking of the Dacron bypass, which resulted in complete occlusion in two of eight animals. To avoid such occurrences, subsequent intraluminal bypass devices were modified to have only one stent at the proximal end. In addition, the Dacron graft was crimped to allow for shortening without kinking. The distal end of the graft was allowed to expand and apply against the aortic wall like a wind sock. Leakage from the distal end of the graft into the excluded aneurysmal lumen was avoided by matching the diameters of the graft and distal aorta. Of five attempted placements of this device for exclusion of an abdominal aortic aneurysm in five patients, four were successful.[9] In the single patient with failed placement because of miscalculation of the graft length, the device was removed surgically and an aortic-bifemoral bypass was performed. A follow-up aortogram obtained in two patients at 10 weeks showed patency of the graft in both. One patient had a small leakage of the distal end of the graft into the excluded aneurysmal lumen, and the aneurysm did not thrombose completely. Longer follow-up and a well-controlled trial will be necessary to establish the safety and efficacy of this new method. Modifications are likely to develop as experience increases.

CURRENT CLINICAL EXPERIENCE WITH INTRAVASCULAR STENTS

Evaluation of the clinical experience with intravascular stents must include data regarding acute occlusion, patency, and complications. Acute occlusion data are important because of the inherent thrombogenicity of these devices. In this respect, most authors agree that thrombotic events occurring within 3 weeks after placement are considered acute occlusions. Patency of the stent lumen may be indicated as minimal luminal diameter or mean percentage of stenosis. However, most commonly, stent patency is expressed as the percentage of stents with a lumen less than or equal to 50% of the postplacement diameter. Regarding the appropriate time of angiographic follow-up, most authors report their experience at 6 months. Complications of stent placement must include those related to the procedure in general and those related to the device itself. Acute thrombotic events must be considered a complication and, therefore, are added to the complication rate.

ILIAC ARTERIES

The use of stents in the iliac arteries is supported by the results of two multicenter trials in the United States and Germany, respectively. The U.S. trial, started in 1987, collectively accumulated 486 patients. The angiographic patency rate was 92% at 8.7 months and the clinical success was 69% at 43 months. The discrepancy was due to the development of new disease distal to the treated site that made itself clinically evident at a rate of 5%/yr. The complication rate of 9.9% was not significantly different from the reported complication rate of percutaneous iliac angioplasty. The German trial, which is still in progress, involves randomization of iliac stenting vs. balloon angioplasty. The clinical success rate of stenting in this trial was 96.6% at 3 years as opposed to 68.3% for angioplasty.

Technical Aspects

The only device currently approved for clinical use in the iliac arteries by the U.S. Food and Drug Administration is the Palmaz stent (Johnson and Johnson Interventional Systems, Warren, NJ). The P308 stent measures 3.1 mm in diameter by 30 mm in length and can be expanded to 12 mm in diameter. The balloon angioplasty catheters recommended to deploy the stent are the USCI-PE Plus II (USCI, Billerica, Mass), Meditech PEMT (Meditech, Watertown, Mass), and Cordis 7F PTA balloon catheter (Cordis Co, Miami, Fla), all of which have a shaft of 7 French, a balloon diameter of 8 mm, and a length of 3 cm. The stent is crimped on the balloon with a crimping tool and is carried to the site of deployment through a 9-French vascular access sheath with a hemostatic valve. The balloon-stent combination is advanced through the valve with the aid of a metal introducer tube, which is removed after the stent is in the sheath lumen. The stent is placed within the target area under fluoroscopic visualization because of the radiopacity of the stent and the balloon markers. Contrast injections through the sidearm of the vascular access sheath help in final positioning of the stent prior to its deployment. After withdrawal of the sheath to expose the stent within the vessel lumen, the balloon is inflated while monitoring the patient's pain response. Following balloon deflation and withdrawal, it is customary to measure pressure gradients and perform an arteriogram through a catheter previously ex-

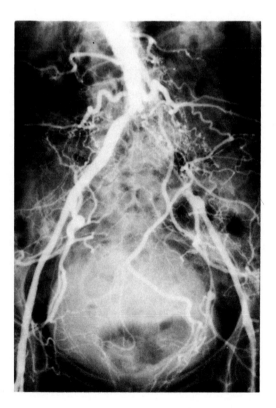

FIGURE 9.

Two stents are deployed simultaneously with their cephalad ends 10 mm inside the aortic stent. Two additional stents completed the recanalization of the left common iliac artery.

changed over the guidewire. Systemic heparinization is used only during the procedure, with an average intravenous dose of 3,000 to 5,000 units. Prolonged heparinization or oral anticoagulation in general is not necessary. To decrease the risk of hematoma at the puncture site, the sheath is pulled out of the femoral artery after the partial thromboplastin time is close to normal. Reversal of the heparinization by protamine is not recommended.

Stenting of long iliac stenoses, dissections, or occlusion requires multiple stents, which may be placed with variable degrees of overlap depending on the length of the arterial segment and the number of stents used (Figs 9 through 14). Vessels larger than 8 mm in diameter require further stent expansion by larger balloons. The balloons are exchanged without difficulty if access to the stent lumen is assured by permanency of the guidewire through the iliac artery and abdominal aorta. The success of the procedure largely depends on initial passage of the guidewire through the lesion. Sometimes, traversing a severe stenosis or occlusion with a probing guidewire requires considerable skill and excellent fluoroscopic visualization. A curved, hydrophilic, coated guidewire such as the 0.035-in. Glidewire (Meditech, Watertown, Mass) is very useful for

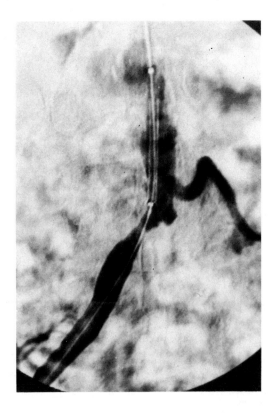

FIGURE 10.

Abdominal aortogram showing chronic occlusion of the left common iliac artery and high-grade stenosis of the origin of the right common iliac artery. The distal aorta is narrowed markedly.

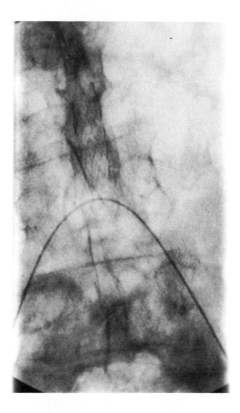

FIGURE 11.

A balloon-mounted P308 Palmaz stent is placed at the distal aorta. Contrast injection defines stent position prior to deployment.

this purpose. However, after reaching the aortic lumen, it is better to exchange this guidewire over a straight 5-French catheter by a stiff 0.035 or 0.038 Amplatz guidewire (Meditech, Watertown, Mass) to avoid kinking of the sheath by bends in the iliac arteries. Even marked tortuosities can be overcome by the use of this guidewire. Preventing kinking of the sheath avoids dislodgments of the stent off the balloon and the possibility of balloon perforation. If this occurs, the balloon must be exchanged after careful advancement of the sheath to the flared end of the incompletely expanded stent. The tip of the sheath helps to stabilize the stent as the perforated balloon is pulled into the sheath lumen. Introduction and inflation of a new balloon completes the stent expansion.

Complex cases may require multiple catheter and guidewire exchanges in substantial modification of the previously described technique. An example of this is the pull-through guidewire access, as illustrated in Figures 9 through 14. This case also illustrates one of the ways to stent the aortic bifurcation by placing "kissing stents" partially inside of a previously placed aortic stent.

A number of applications of stents have been made outside of the iliac arteries. Some of them are under protocol investigation and others have been exceptional "off-label" uses of the iliac stent. The following is a brief description of these uses and their results.

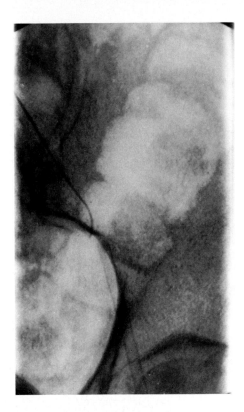

FIGURE 12.
Due to failure to advance a guidewire through the left femoral sheath retrogradely, a guidewire is advanced antegradely across the bifurcation.

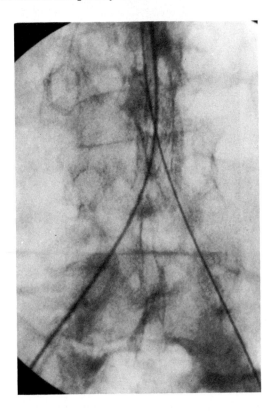

FIGURE 13.
The wire is introduced into the left femoral sheath and exteriorized through the valve.

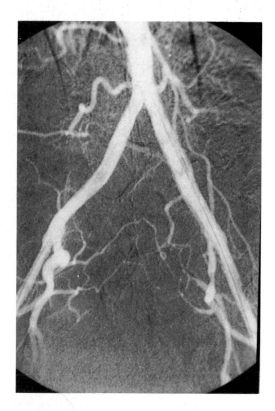

FIGURE 14.

Guidewires finally are placed bilaterally through both femoral sheaths and across the distal aortic stent.

FEMOROPOPLITEAL ARTERIES

Experience with stent placement in the femoropopliteal arteries with the Palmaz stent largely comes from France. The collective experience of two centers in this country is encouraging. Acute thrombotic events occurred in 5% of the cases. The 6-month patency rate was 86% and the complication rate was 9%. The collective experience from two German and one Swiss centers with the Wallstent in this application indicated a rate of 21.5% of acute thrombosis, a patency rate of 68.5%, and a complication rate of 26%. However, the results with these two stents cannot be compared directly because of dissimilar patient selection. Most of the lesions treated with the Palmaz stent were shorter than those treated with the Wallstent.

Technical Aspects

Current experience suggests that superficial femoral artery stenting should be limited to lesions shorter than 6 cm that have significant elastic recoil or flow-limiting dissection following balloon angioplasty. The segment of the superficial femoral artery that is amenable to stenting extends from 5 cm below the femoral ligament to the adductor canal. Stenting of this artery requires downhill placement of a femoral sheath. The Wallstent may be introduced from the opposite groin in the absence of iliac artery disease. Generally, a 7-French sheath is necessary to intro-

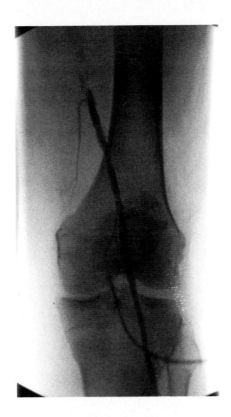

FIGURE 15.
Inability to cross a left distal superficial femoral artery occlusion motivates a percutaneous popliteal retrograde approach.

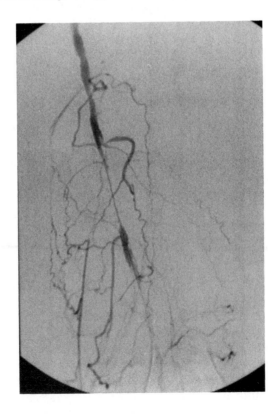

FIGURE 16.
A guidewire is advanced easily across the 2-cm-long occlusion, into the proximal true lumen.

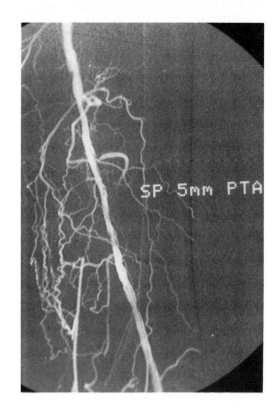

FIGURE 17.
Arteriogram following preliminary dilatation with a 5-mm balloon.

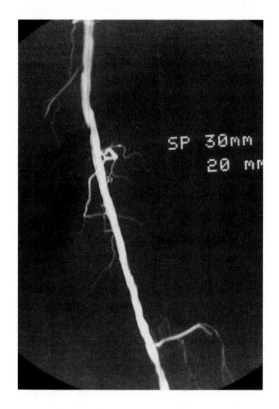

FIGURE 18.
Arteriogram following placement of a P-294 and a P-204 Palmaz stent. Stents were mounted on 6-mm, 5-French balloons.

duce the Palmaz 294 stent crimped on a Meditech PEMT-5, 5- to 7-mm balloon. As with stenting of iliac artery disease, the success of the procedure depends on successful probing of the lesion by a guidewire. Short-segment occlusions may be treated previously with a short period of fibrinolytic infusion using the pulse-spray technique. Inability to cross the lesion antegradely may require a retrograde popliteal artery approach (Figs 15 to 18). Femoral stenting necessitates oral anticoagulation for 3 to 6 months.

RENAL ARTERIES

The collective experience with placement of Palmaz-Schatz stents in renal arteries showed a patency rate of 77%, no acute thrombotic occlusions, and a complication rate of 9%. European trials with the Wallstent demonstrated an average patency rate of 82.1%, acute thrombosis in 7.1%, and a 25% complication rate. The results of renal artery stenting with these two devices cannot be compared directly, as most of the patients treated with the Palmaz-Schatz stent had ostial renal artery stenosis, whereas less than half of those receiving the Wallstent were in this category.

Technical Aspects

Placement of a straight Palmaz or an articulated Palmaz-Schatz stent requires the insertion of an 8-French introducer sheath in the groin. Preferably, this sheath should be 25 cm long to avoid damaging the iliac artery or the aortic bifurcation during catheter exchanges. The stent is crimped on a Meditech PEMT-5 or Ultrathin ST (Meditech, Watertown, Mass) balloon 5 to 7 mm in diameter by 2 cm in length and is backloaded in a wide-lumen 8-French hockey-stick guide catheter such as the Cordis peripheral guiding catheter (0.084-in. internal diameter; Cordis Co., Miami, Fla) attached to a hemostatic valve adaptor. The system is introduced into the renal artery over a 0.035-in., 180-cm-long Rosen guidewire (Cook, Inc., Bloomington, Ind) following predilation of the lesion with a balloon 2 mm smaller than the desired stent diameter. As with iliac and femoral lesions, successful crossing of the lesion with a guidewire is critical. This usually is accomplished with a 0.035 angled-tip Glidewire and a cobra-2 or Simmons catheter (Meditech, Watertown, Mass). After the catheter tip is advanced past the stenotic area, the probing guidewire can be exchanged for the small "J" Rosen guidewire (Cook, Inc., Bloomington, Ind) for angioplasty and stenting. These manipulations require intravenous heparinization (5,000 to 10,000 units) and intrarenal nitroglycerin in boluses of 100 to 200 μg. The precise positioning of the stent is aided by contrast injections under fluoroscopic control through the sidearm of the hemostatic valve attached to the guidecatheter. The stent is deployed with its aortic end flush with the aortic lumen. When using selected frames from digital arteriograms obtained prior to deployment, it is essential that they be obtained in the exact same axial angulation of the "C" arm as the one used during deployment, to avoid parallax errors. This may result in miscalculation of the ostium site and placement of the stent too far into the renal artery or partially in the aortic lumen.

LARGE VEINS

The largest experience with stenting in the large veins was reported with the Gianturco "Z" stent. Most of the applications of this device were in patients with advanced neoplastic disease and superior or inferior vena cava obstruction. In a large percentage of the patients, the symptoms are palliated with an acceptable complication rate, considering the severe nature of the disease treated. The small experience with the Palmaz stent and the Wallstent is encouraging also. The patency rate obtained in patients with dialysis shunts and central vein stenosis parallels the poor results obtained with balloon angioplasty in this setting. Whether stent placement is beneficial to prolong the life of access shunts must await further evaluation.

Technical Aspects

The most common venous occlusion requiring the use of stent recanalization is superior vena cava syndrome (Figs 19 and 20). In general, when symptoms are present, extensive thrombosis of the innominate, jugular, and subclavian veins is detected on the preliminary studies. This requires

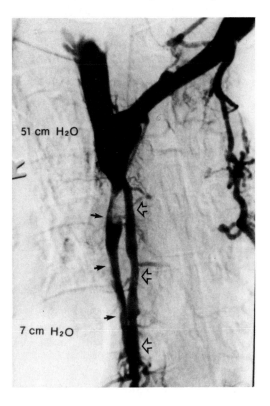

FIGURE 19.

Contrast injection at the confluence of the innominate veins in a patient with superior vena cava syndrome and advanced lung neoplasm. The superior vena cava is encased to the point of almost complete occlusion (*arrows*). The azygous vein (*arrowheads*) provides collateral flow to inferior vena cava tributaries. Pressure gradient was 44 cm of saline.

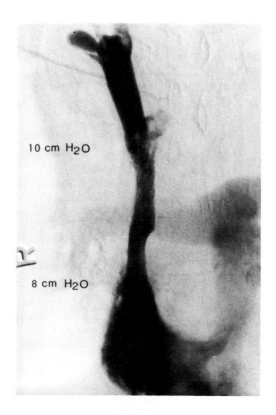

FIGURE 20.

A single PS-30 Palmaz stent provides adequate flow through the superior vena cava. The stent was dilated to 10 mm in diameter. Pressure gradient was reduced to 2 cm of saline.

fibrinolysis followed by guidewire probing of the neoplastic obstruction. Stents may be introduced via the femoral or brachial veins through a 9-French access sheath, over a stiff guidewire. Several stents may be required to obtain adequate recanalization of the superior vena cava and the final diameter may be a compromise between acceptable flow and the patient's pain during stent deployment. As with the iliac arteries, judicious expansion of the stent must take into account pain sensation as the only way to monitor distensibility of the vascular structure within elastic limits. Often, not all inferior tributaries of the superior vena cava can be recanalized in cases of extensive venous thrombosis. However, symptomatic relief often is obtained with recanalization of just either one of the subclavian or jugular veins.

TRANSJUGULAR, INTRAHEPATIC, PORTOSYSTEMIC STENT SHUNT

Transjugular, intrahepatic, portosystemic stent shunt (TIPSS) is a new form of percutaneous therapy to achieve portal vein decompression in patients with portal hypertension. It is based on the creation of a conduit between the portal vein or one of its main branches and a hepatic vein through interposed liver parenchyma. The technique consists of progressive dilatation of a needle track with balloon angioplasty catheters followed by the placement of metallic stents. The procedure requires thorough operator training, state-of-the-art angiographic radiographic equipment, and a wide selection of catheters and needles. However, the method is well established and the shunt can be accomplished within 2 to 3 hours in most patients. Because of the relatively low invasiveness of this form of therapy, it may be applied to critically ill patients in whom other forms of therapy have failed to control and severe consequences of portal hypertension and advanced liver disease. The major challenge in the application of this form of therapy other than mastering the technique is in the handling of preprocedural and postprocedural care. In addition to providing portal decompression to patients who cannot afford general anesthesia and abdominal surgery, the potential benefit of TIPSS relates to savings in blood and blood products, and to the prevention of prolonged stays in the intensive care unit.

Early clinical experience was obtained at the University of Freiburg in three patients with life-threatening variceal hemorrhage and severe chronic liver disease.[10] The procedure was technically successful in all three patients and involved the use of a combined transjugular and percutaneous transhepatic approach. The latter allowed the use of a wire basket serving as a target for directing the needle tip to the portal entry site. One of the patients, who had severe hepatorenal failure, died of adult respiratory distress syndrome 11 days after the procedure. The other two survived without further bleeding, and portograms at 6 months demonstrated patent shunts and adequate portal decompression.

Further clinical experience at the Freiburg and Heidelberg university clinics yielded substantial refinements of the technique and improvements in patient management.[11] Of 59 attempts at TIPSS, 53 were technically successful. Of these 53 patients (average age, 61 years), 42 had alcoholic and 17 had postnecrotic liver cirrhosis. Twenty-one patients had Child's C, 29 had Child's B, and 9 had Child's A metabolic status. Shunting resulted in a 52% reduction of the portal pressure. Immediate complications included one episode of lethal intraperitoneal bleeding following withdrawal of the transhepatic catheter among the early experiences. Within 1 month after TIPSS, all 53 patients had a patent shunt. Thirty-day mortality included two additional deaths (6%). Recurrent gastrointestinal bleeding occurred in 4 patients, but no evidence of encephalopathy was encountered in the first 30 days. Long-term observation averaged 14 months (range, 2 to 39 months). Angiographic and/or Doppler ultrasound examination was performed every 6 months, demonstrating a patent shunt in 49 patients at the latest follow-up. Late mortality amounts to 19%, with one death related to shunt thrombosis and recurrent variceal bleeding. Two additional patients developed late gastrointestinal hemorrhage and 4 developed encephalopathy.

It was the conclusion of the authors that the procedure was safe and effective, and that it was indicated in patients with advanced liver disease and uncorrectable coagulopathy. It also was deemed adequate for patients with failed surgical portosystemic shunt and for those awaiting liver transplantation.

Similar conclusions regarding safety and effectiveness were reached by the group at the Miami Vascular Institute. Zemel and coworkers[12] gathered preliminary experience in 8 patients with a history of esophageal variceal bleeding and portal hypertension. TIPSS decreased the average portal pressure from 36 to 11 mm Hg. Complications included migration of a stent from the shunt site to a pulmonary artery. The migrated stent was withdrawn into the inferior vena cava bifurcation and deployed there by further balloon expansion. Another patient had recurrent hemorrhoidal bleeding that necessitated further lowering of the portal pressure by additional shunt dilatation. Upper gastrointestinal endoscopy performed routinely 1 week following the procedure demonstrated collapse of the gastroesophageal varices. In 2 patients, severe ascites was reduced to trace amounts, and in 4 additional patients, moderate ascites was resolved completely. None of the patients developed encephalopathy. The average hospital stay was 7.7 (range, 1 to 19) days.

At the University of Texas Health Science Center at San Antonio, the emphasis with TIPSS is focused on patients with active, life-threatening hemorrhage who do not respond to intravenous vasopressin (Pitressin) infusion, endoscopic sclerotherapy, and placement of a gastroesophageal balloon. Thirty-nine patients, with an average age of 49.3 ± 11.6 years, were in this category. Of these, 36 had active esophageal or gastric variceal bleeding and 3 had spontaneous intraperitoneal bleeding. Thirteen patients had postnecrotic cirrhosis, 7 had alcoholic liver disease, and 9 had liver cirrhosis of undetermined etiology. According to the Child's ranking system, 21 patients were in the C category, 15 were in the B category, and 3 were in the A category. The severe clinical status of these patients was reflected by their requirements of an average of 18.5 ± 16 units of blood or blood products during this hospital admission.

The average portal pressure of 46 ± 10 cm of saline and the portosystemic gradient of 27 ± 12 cm of saline prior to TIPSS were reduced after treatment to 37 ± 13 and 7 ± 4 cm of saline, respectively. TIPSS reduced the average blood transfusion requirement to 1 unit prior to discharge or death. Thirty-day mortality was high in this group of patients (10 of 39, 26%) and included fatalities from heart failure, adult respiratory distress syndrome, and sepsis. Shunt patency as established by routine 1-week portal catheterization or autopsy among the fatalities was 100%. Mean blood ammonia was 68 mOsm/L before TIPSS, 64 mOsm/L at 1 week after TIPSS, and 69 mOsm/L at 2 weeks after TIPSS. These preliminary results are quite encouraging, taking into consideration the poor clinical status of these patients. This early experience will require further evaluation, including randomization studies, in order to define its role and indications, and to assess its effectiveness and safety.

Technical Aspects

In preparation for the procedure, we attempt to correct coagulation disorders and serum albumin deficits. Portal and hepatic venous anatomy and pressures are documented by arterial portogram and transcatheter venography on a date prior to the TIPSS procedure in nonemergent situations. The right internal jugular vein is cannulated percutaneously and access is established by placement of a 10-French, 30-cm-long sheath with a hemostatic valve (Cook Inc., Bloomington, Ind), with the tip in the proximal portion of the vein. A modified Ross needle (Cook, Inc., Bloomington, Ind) or a Richter needle (Angiomed, Karlsruhe, Germany) protected

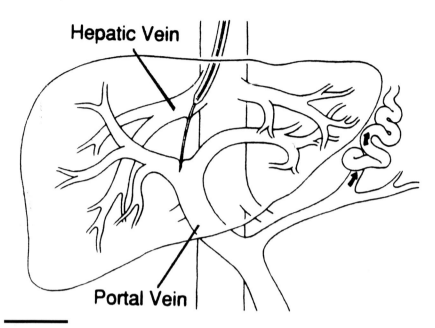

FIGURE 21.

Schematic representation of a needle entering the portal vein bifurcation through the proximal middle hepatic vein by the transjugular approach. (From Zemel G, Katzen BT, et al: *JAMA* 1991; 266:390–393. Used by permission.)

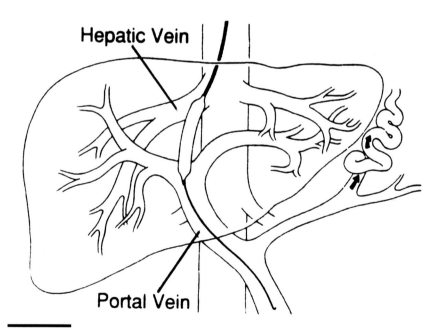

FIGURE 22.

A balloon is expanded in the parenchymal needle track.

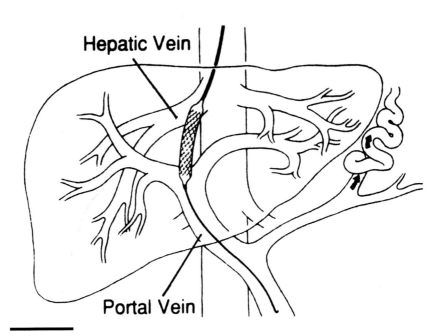

FIGURE 23.

A balloon-expandable stent is deployed within the track.

with a Teflon sleeve is advanced past the tip of the sheath. The needle tip is aimed anteromedially under fluoroscopy with the guidance of the needle's hub indicator. After aiming the tip of the needle to the lower aspect of the proximal portion of the hepatic vein, the sleeve is retracted, exposing the tip, and it is advanced caudally. Considerable resistance is

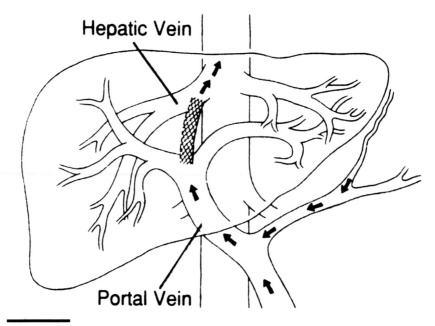

FIGURE 24.

Following balloon deflation and withdrawal, flow is established through the shunt.

met in most patients due to advanced periportal fibrosis. Entrance into
the portal vein lumen usually is felt as a sudden give with a tactile "pop"
(Fig 21). If blood is aspirated from the needle lumen and a hand injection of contrast material confirms intraportal position, a heavy-duty 0.035-
in. guidewire (Amplatz Extra-stiff, Cook Inc., Bloomington, Ind) is advanced past the superior mesenteric vein and into one of its branches.
The needle tract first is dilated by advancing the protective sleeve of the
needle over the guidewire.

Following removal of the needle and sleeve, an 8-mm balloon angioplasty catheter (UT 8×3, Meditech, Watertown, Mass) is introduced over
the wire, positioned within the tract, and inflated (Fig 22). The profile of
the balloon opacified with diluted contrast generally indicates where the
portal and hepatic vein walls are by localized constrictions or "waists"
at less than maximal inflation pressure. These are important landmarks
for the placement of stents because they represent points of high recoil
that must be scaffolded securely by the stent. This is achieved by placing
the stents at least 1 cm within the portal vein and hepatic vein lumens.
After deflation and withdrawal of the angioplasty balloon, the sheath is
advanced with its dilator within the track. The dilator then is replaced
by the stent (PS-30, Johnson and Johnson Interventional Systems, War-

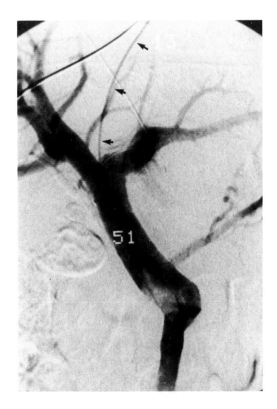

FIGURE 25.

Portogram following transjugular access. The needle was exchanged by a
5-French catheter for contrast injection and manometry (*arrows*). The right
atrial pressure was measured through the sidearm of the transjugular sheath.
The portosystemic gradient was 38 cm of saline.

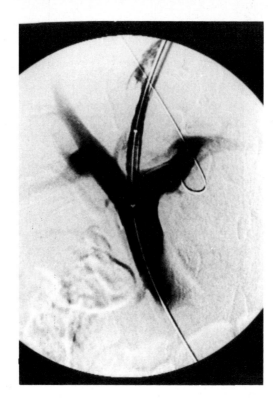

FIGURE 26.
A stent is positioned in the parenchymal track previously dilated by a balloon.

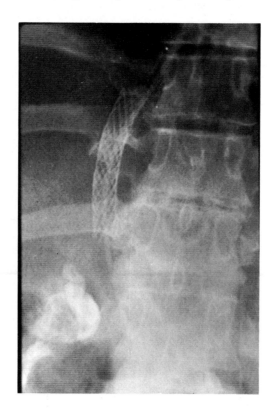

FIGURE 27.
Two stents are placed tandem to cover the parenchymal track.

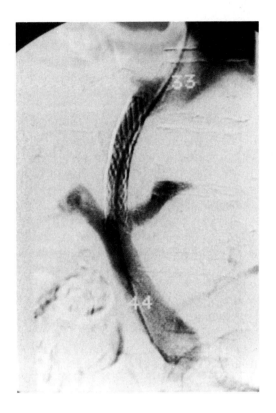

FIGURE 28.

Portogram after transjugular, intrahepatic, portosystemic stent shunt. Good flow is observed through the shunt. The portosystemic gradient fell to 11 cm of saline.

ren, NJ) crimped on a high-pressure balloon (PE-Plus 8×3, USCI, Billerica, Mass; Fig 23). Contrast injections through the sidearm of the sheath allow precise positioning of the stents in relation to the track. The distal stent is deployed first after withdrawal of the sheath (Fig 24). Most commonly, a second stent and, on occasion, a third, are necessary to cover the whole tract, depending on its length. After the balloon is deflated and exchanged by an angiographic catheter, contrast injection and manometry indicate whether further expansion of shunt is necessary to achieve adequate portal decompression (see Fig 24).

Following positioning of an angiographic straight 5-French catheter with multiple sideholes in the proximal splenic vein, contrast injection at a rate of 10 cc/sec for 3 to 4 sec should be adequate to evaluate properly the direction of the blood flow in the left gastric vein and other portosystemic collaterals (Figs 25 to 28). If adequate decompression is achieved, flow in the collaterals should be in the direction of the portal vein. In general, following an effective shunt, blood flow in the portal branches is diminished greatly, preventing their opacification. Although there is no fast rule regarding the ideal portohepatic gradient, more than 20 cm of saline should be an indication for further shunt dilatation. This can be accomplished readily by introducing a 9 to 12 mm × 4 cm balloon angioplasty catheter. Larger balloons have an increased tendency to get tethered inside of the shunt because of the larger "wings" of the deflated balloon. Therefore, the catheter must be manipulated carefully to prevent disruption of the shunt or dislodgment of balloon material. The use of the Olbert balloon (Meadox-Surgimed Inc., Oakland, NJ), which does not have wings after deflation, may represent an advantage in this respect.

The role of concomitant embolization of the portosystemic collaterals is not clear, and some authors believe that it is not necessary if adequate decompression is achieved.[12] We found it useful to embolize the left gastric vein after TIPSS in patients with severe coagulopathy and active bleeding in order to expedite the removal of the gastroesophageal balloon and to stop the vasopressin infusion.

The intraoperative management of the patient depends on whether TIPSS is performed electively or emergently. Under elective conditions, the patient is sedated only mildly to obtain maximum cooperation with regard to holding respiration, changes in position, and pain monitoring. Physiologic monitoring usually is limited to automated cuff blood pressure recording, pulse oximetry, and electrocardiographic tracing. In critically ill patients, it is advisable also to have direct arterial pressure monitoring and a Swan-Ganz catheter with thermodilution capability in place. Agitated patients may need more profound sedation and, therefore, closer monitoring. Actively bleeding patients pose additional challenge because the angiographic laboratory, already crowded with monitoring equipment, nursing, and technical aids, must meet the sterile precautions necessary for the implantation of foreign vascular material.

REFERENCES

1. Dotter CT: Transluminally-placed coilspring endarterial tube grafts. Long-term patency in canine popliteal artery. *Invest Radiol* 1969; 4:329–332.
2. Sauvage LR: Externally supported, noncrimped external velour, weft-knitted Dacron prostheses for axillofemoral, femoropopliteal, and femorotibial bypass, in Wright CB, Hosson RW, Hiratzka LF, et al (eds): *Vascular Grafting: Clinical Applications and Techniques.* Boston, Wright, 1983, pp 158–186.
3. Palmaz JC, Garcia O, Kopp DT, et al: Balloon-expandable intraarterial stents: Effect of antithrombotic medication on thrombus formation, in Zeitler E (ed): *Pros and Cons in PTA and Auxiliary Methods.* New York, Springer Verlag, 1989, pp 170–178.
4. Palmaz JC: Balloon-expandable intravascular stent. *AJR Am J Roentgenol* 1988; 150:1263–1269.
5. Noeldge G, Richter GM, Siegestetter V, et al: Tierexperimentelle Untersuchungen uber den Einflub der Flubrestriktion auf die Thrombogenitat des Palmaz Stentes mittels 111-Indium-markierter Thrombozyten. *ROFO* 1990; 152:264–270.
6. Palmaz JC, Tio FO, Schatz RA, et al: Early endothelisation of balloon-expandable stents: Experimental observations. *J Intervent Radiol* 1988; 3:119–124.
7. Dichek DA, Neville RF, Zwiebel JA, et al: Seeding of intravascular stents with genetically engineered endothelial cells. *Circulation* 1989; 80:1347–1353.
8. Laborde JC, Parodi JC, Clem MF, et al: Intraluminal bypass of abdominal aortic aneurysm: A feasibility study. *Radiology* 1992; 184:185–190.

9. Parodi JC, Palmaz JC, Barone HD: Transfemoral intraluminal graft: Implantation for abdominal aortic aneurysms. *Ann Vasc Surg* 1991; S491–499.

10. Richter GM, Noeldge G, Palmaz JC, et al: Transjugular intrahepatic portacaval stent shunt: Preliminary clinical results. *Radiology* 1990; 174:1027–1030.

11. Richter GM, Noeldge G, Roessle M, et al: Three-year results of use of transjugular intrahepatic portosystemic stent shunt (abstract). *Radiology* 1991; 181:99.

12. Zemel G, Katzen BT, Becker GJ, et al: Percutaneous transjugular portosystemic shunt. *JAMA* 1991; 266:390–393.

Intraluminal Ultrasound and the Management of Peripheral Vascular Disease

DOUGLAS M. CAVAYE, M.B., B.S., F.R.A.C.S.

RODNEY A. WHITE, M.D.

Intraluminal ultrasound (ILUS) has developed rapidly during the last 5 years, and it provides a unique perspective from which to view vascular disease and the effects of intervention. ILUS uses combined advances in catheter technology, echographic data processing, and computerized image manipulation to produce accurate luminal and transmural images of blood vessels. Although these devices have been available only for a relatively short time, numerous diagnostic and therapeutic applications have been reported and proposed (Table 1). A major thrust of current ILUS development is its application as an adjunct to peripheral angioplasty procedures and incorporation into endovascular therapeutic catheters. By providing a detailed image of vessels before, during, and after intervention, ILUS provides a method for both guidance of endoluminal devices and immediate assessment of the results of the procedure. These capabilities are applicable to therapeutic techniques, including balloon angioplasty, mechanical atherectomy, laser-assisted angioplasty, and intravascular stent development. In addition to playing a pivotal role in the development of newer, more effective endovascular devices, ILUS offers exciting possibilities in peripheral vascular research such as investigation of blood vessel compliance and dynamic changes in the vessel wall caused by disease or pharmacologic intervention, and elucidation of the morphologic changes associated with the natural history of atherosclerosis.

INTRALUMINAL ULTRASOUND IMAGING DEVICES

A major advantage of transcutaneous (i.e., duplex) ultrasound imaging over arteriography is its painless, noninvasive nature. In addition to avoiding radiographic contrast agents and ionizing radiation, it does not require invasive access to the patient's vessels. Why, therefore, use an ILUS device? Transcutaneous ultrasound imaging suffers from various limitations related to image data acquisition, despite recent refinements

Advances in Vascular Surgery, vol. 1.
©1993, Mosby–Year Book, Inc.

TABLE 1.

Applications of Intraluminal Ultrasound

I. Diagnostic.
   A. Demonstrate luminal shape and disease location.
      1. Eccentric vs. concentric lumen.
      2. Display luminal ellipticity.
      3. Differentiate aortic stenosis vs. coarctation.
   B. Determine vessel cross-sectional dimensions.
      1. Accurately measure percent luminal stenosis.
      2. Quantitate medial and intimal thickening.
   C. Tissue characterization.
      1. Identify plaque composition (lipid, smooth muscle cell, fibrous, calcium).
      2. Differentiate plaque from thrombus.
   D. Arterial dissection.
      1. Identify dissection entry site and locate flap.
      2. Determine false lumen relationship to major branch orifices.
   E. Identify and localize intravascular tumors.
II. Therapeutic.
   A. Match interventional method with lesion characteristic.
   B. Elucidate mechanisms of angioplasty.
      1. Quantitate wall stretching, dissection, plaque rupture.
      2. Assess recoil and spasm, need for further intervention.
   C. Guide angioplasty devices.
      1. Aid selection of device size (balloon, atherectomy burr).
      2. Guide endoluminal ablation devices (i.e., lasers).
   D. Assess effects of therapy.
      1. Real-time intraluminal imaging of balloon angioplasty.
      2. Measure plaque and lumen areas preintervention and postintervention.
      3. Provide accurate control data.
   E. Aid intravascular stent deployment.
      1. Assess primary intervention (i.e., is a stent required?).
      2. Stent positioning, size selection.
      3. Confirmation of deployment.

that have expanded its diagnostic capabilities to the visceral and cerebral circulations. In general, deep vascular structures or those obscured by bone or lung are not well seen, leading investigators to develop innovative methods of intracorporeal ultrasound. By attaching the transducer to an intraluminal catheter, the imaging elements could be placed much closer to the target structure. As a result, the use of higher-frequency ultrasound (up to 50 MHz) became practical, since the problem of increased attenuation of the energy by subcutaneous or other intervening tissue was overcome by the proximity of the transducer to the imaged structure. Both of these features produced great improvements in image quality, and the noninvasive nature of transcutaneous ultrasound was traded effectively for improved resolution of deep-lying or poorly accessible structures.

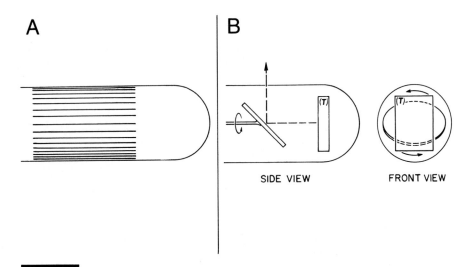

FIGURE 1.

A, electronically switched array with multiple transducer elements placed circumferentially. **B,** mechanical device using a fixed transducer (T) and proximally
placed rotating acoustic mirror. Both types of device produce a 360-degree, cross-
sectional image of the blood vessel.

INTRAVASCULAR CROSS-SECTIONAL IMAGING

A 360-degree, cross-sectional image is obtained by scanning the ultrasound beam through a full circle and synchronizing the beam direction
and deflection with the display. This is achieved either by mechanically
rotating the imaging elements, or by using electronically switched arrays
(Fig 1).

Electronically Switched Arrays

A number of individual elements (e.g., 64) using frequencies of 15 to 30
MHz are placed circumferentially at the tip of a catheter along with a miniaturized integrated circuit, resulting in sequenced transmission and re-
ception by the imaging elements in groups. These catheters usually are
more flexible than mechanical devices, but they suffer from poor imaging in the close near-field because the imaging crystals are only a very
short distance from the surrounding blood or tissue. A bright circumferential artifact known as the "ring down" or "halo" obscures structures in
the vicinity of the catheter border, despite the use of gain-compensation
and suppression techniques. Electronically switched array catheters can
be constructed with a central lumen suitable for a centrally placed
guidewire, whereas rotating mechanical devices require a coaxial mono-
rail configuration. In small vessels, or following intervention where there
may be medial dissection, a centrally placed guidewire may be advanta-
geous when advancing the ILUS catheter.

Mechanical Transducers

There are two basic configurations: (1) the transducer is rotated at the tip
of the catheter, or (2) an acoustic mirror is rotated that deflects the ultrasound beam produced by a distally placed, fixed transducer. In both types
of devices, ultrasound frequencies of 10 to 30 MHz are used, although

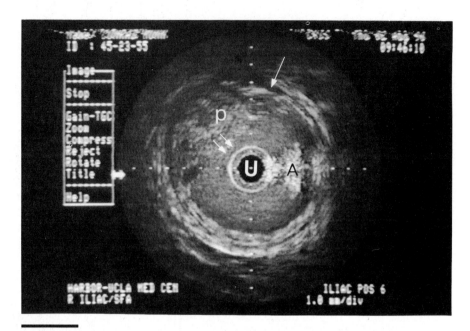

FIGURE 2.

Intraluminal ultrasound image of a human iliac artery. The transducer artifact *(A)* obscures about 15 degrees of the circumference of the image. Ultrasound catheter void *(U)*, normal vessel wall *(arrow)*, soft plaque *(p)*, and plaque/lumen interface *(double arrows)* are seen. (From Tabbara MR, White RA, Cavaye DM, et al: *J Vasc Surg* 1991; 14:496–502. Used by permission.)

some experimental catheters using frequencies up to 45 MHz or higher have produced excellent images of human vessels in vitro.[1] An advantage of the rotating mirror device is the distance that it requires between the transducer and the deflecting mirror, which virtually eliminates the halo artifact, since the immediate near-field is comprised of echolucent saline in the imaging assembly chamber. The scan converter in the image processing unit compensates for this nonimaging portion of the beam and generates images beginning precisely at the border of the catheter. Also, an electrical connecting wire passes along the side of the imaging chamber, producing an artifact that occupies 15 degrees of the cross-sectional image (Fig 2).

THREE-DIMENSIONAL COMPUTERIZED IMAGE RECONSTRUCTION

Algorithms of three-dimensional (3D) image reconstruction can be classified as either surface- or volume-rendering. Currently available 3D ILUS imaging uses surface rendering, in which object surfaces are formed prior to creation of the image on a two-dimensional (2D) screen using methods such as hidden-part removal, shading, dynamic rotation, and stereo projection.[2] In summary, a longitudinally aligned set (up to 450 images per set) of consecutive 2D ILUS images is "stacked" in sequence to produce the 3D image (Fig 3). The 2D images are acquired by slowly withdrawing the catheter through the vessel segment at a uniform rate, either manually or using a mechanical device. This "pullback" can be recorded on tape or reconstructed on-line following analogue-to-digital conversion

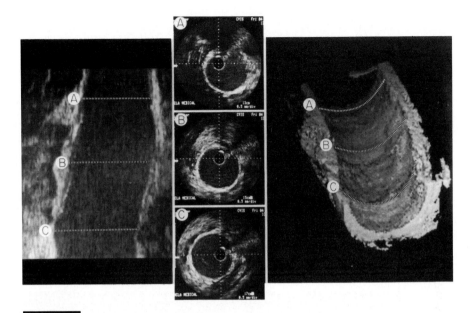

FIGURE 3.

Principle of computerized intraluminal ultrasound image reconstruction. The two-dimensional images labeled *A, B,* and *C (center panel)* are "stacked" by the computer, and correspond to the sites labeled with the same letter on the three-dimensional image *(right)* and on the longitudinal section of the three-dimensional image *(left)*. (From Cavaye DM, Tabbara MR, Kopchok GE, et al: *Am Surg* 1991; 57:751–755. Used by permission.)

and frame sampling at rates up to 30 frames per second. The initial step in image processing produces a real-time, gray-scale, longitudinal section of the vessel that can be rotated through 360 degrees to facilitate interrogation of specific sites. Additional computer processing time of about 20 seconds is required to produce a 3D rendered image that can be manipulated on-screen and allow examination from any user-defined projection.

FORWARD-LOOKING INTRALUMINAL ULTRASOUND

An exciting recent advance is the development of forward-looking ILUS, using acoustic beams that radiate in the shape of a cone from the front of a 7.5-French catheter (Fig 4). A 27-MHz transducer fills a 60-degree divergent cone with 2,000 sequential beams, each comprised of 64 axially aligned acoustic measurements. The result is a 3D image of a volume shaped like a truncated cone, with the near surface located 5 mm from the catheter tip and extending forward 9 mm to the most distant surface. Although this system is experimental, it provides new and unique imaging data that may be critical for guidance of endoluminal devices in treating occlusive vascular lesions.

INTRALUMINAL ULTRASOUND IMAGING TECHNIQUES

VASCULAR ACCESS

ILUS catheters can be introduced either percutaneously or through an incision made in a vessel (arteriotomy or venotomy). Percutaneous access

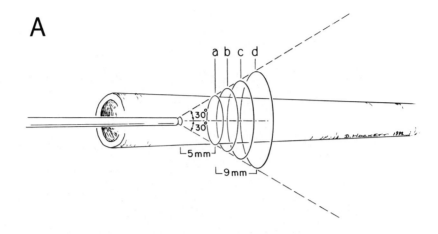

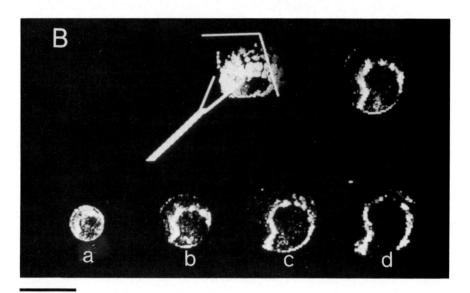

FIGURE 4.

A, schematic representation of forward-looking intraluminal ultrasound catheter. The transducer fills a 60-degree cone with 2,000 sequential beams, resulting in an image shaped like a truncated cone, with the near surface located 5 mm from the catheter tip and the far surface extending back a total of 14 mm. **B,** display screen showing the volume image, catheter icon and cursor above (*upper left*) and representative cross-sections below (*a,b,c,d*). (From Cavaye DM, White RA: *Intravascular Ultrasound Imaging.* New York, Raven Press, 1992, p 107. Used by permission.)

is achieved most commonly using a double-wall arterial puncture, guidewire insertion, and indwelling 8- to 10-French sheath. A single-wall puncture is advisable for patients requiring high femoral puncture (to avoid retroperitoneal hematoma), for patients with a coagulopathy, or for puncture of synthetic grafts. In most situations, a retrograde femoral puncture provides access to the entire aorta and aortoiliac segments using a flexible, 125-cm-long ILUS catheter. It is possible to pass some currently available ILUS catheters via a femoral artery puncture and guidewire control over the aortic bifurcation to the contralateral iliac and lower-limb vessels. However, access to the infralinguinal vessels is achieved best through an antegrade femoral puncture, particularly if a therapeutic intervention is planned. Percutaneous brachial puncture provides access to upper-limb vessels and may be safer and more convenient for imaging thoracoabdominal aortic pathology (e.g., dissection).

Open vascular access is appropriate if ILUS imaging is performed in conjunction with, or as an integral part of, a surgical procedure or open endovascular intervention. Vascular control using circumferential tapes allows atraumatic insertion of the ILUS device, but if multiple or repeated catheter access is required, a hemostatic intraluminal sheath may be used to prevent catheter tip and intimal damage, and to reduce blood loss.

OPTIMIZING IMAGE QUALITY

Intravascular catheter manipulation requires some basic skills, especially when using relatively fragile ILUS catheters via a remote vascular access site. Careful positioning of the imaging tip within the lumen and appropriate size matching of the device to the artery caliber are essential to optimizing visualization. Image quality is best when the catheter is parallel to the vessel axis (i.e., the ultrasound beam is directed at a 90-degree angle to the luminal surface). Minor angulations may affect the luminal shape and dimensional accuracy, whereas eccentric positioning may result in artifactual differences in vessel wall thickness. Careful centering is especially difficult in tortuous vessels, and rotational alignment can be lost as the catheter meanders through the lumen. Several devices can be passed over a guidewire (0.009 to 0.038 in. in diameter), which allows more controlled maneuvering in this situation or in tightly stenotic vessels. As with angioscopy, the best-quality image often is obtained as the catheter is withdrawn, rather than during advancement, since the slight longitudinal tension straightens the catheter and the distal tip tends to find the center of the lumen. Manual rotation of the catheter or external pressure applied to the limb (in extremity-vessel imaging) helps center the transducer. Rotational alignment is achieved by using the image interference artifact as a landmark, and by establishing correct orientation at the site of catheter insertion. The small wire connection that crosses the imaging chamber in most mechanical transducers produces a visual artifact that can be aligned rotationally with an external mark on the catheter and the vessel lumen.

When using mechanical devices, the catheter lumen and guidewire channel must be syringe-flushed manually with saline or water and irrigated continuously with a low-volume, low-pressure system to ensure a bubble-free fluid medium. A problem that results from the use of high-frequency ultrasound and short imaging ranges is the echogenicity of the blood that surrounds the intravascular catheter. Although image preprocessing and postprocessing reduces this phenomenon, special techniques such as luminal flushing with saline or contrast agent may enhance acoustic interfaces dramatically.

IMAGE INTERPRETATION

Distinct sonographic layers are visible in muscular arteries, with the media appearing as an echolucent layer sandwiched between the more echodense intima and adventitia. The exact correlation between the ultrasound image and the microscopic anatomy of the muscular artery wall is still uncertain, although the internal and external elastic laminae and adventitia are considered to be the backscatter substrates for the inner and outer echodense zones.[3] Gussenhoven and colleagues have described four basic plaque components that can be distinguished using a 40-MHz intravascular ultrasound in vitro[3]: (1) echolucent—lipid deposit, lipid "lake"; (2) soft echoes—fibromuscular tissue, intimal proliferation, including varying amounts of diffusely dispersed lipid; (3) bright echoes— collagen-rich fibrous tissue; and (4) bright echoes with acoustic shadowing—calcified tissue. Even small intimal lesions such as flaps or intimal tears are well visualized because of their high fibrous tissue content and the difference in echoic properties of these structures when compared with surrounding blood. The three-layer appearance of muscular arteries is not seen readily in larger vessels (e.g., aorta) because of the increased elastin content in the media.

Several studies have reported that ILUS is accurate in determining the luminal and vessel wall morphology of arteries both in vitro and in vivo, with dimensional accuracy of 0.05 mm.[4-6] The cross-sectional areas calculated from biplanar angiograms and measured from intravascular ultrasound correlate well for normal or minimally diseased peripheral arteries in vivo. Most studies reveal that intravascular ultrasound and angiography also correlate well when used to image mildly elliptical lumina, but when used to derive dimensions from severely diseased vessels, the angiogram tends to underestimate the severity of disease. Precise measurements of the adventitia may be difficult to obtain unless the vessel is surrounded by tissues of differing echogenicity (e.g., echolucent fat).

CLINICAL APPLICATIONS OF INTRALUMINAL ULTRASOUND

The clinical utility of ILUS in the management of peripheral vascular disease can be classified into four primary applications: (1) defining the transmural distribution of disease, (2) characterizing plaque types and intimal lesions, (3) guiding endovascular devices, and (4) providing accurate dimensional data regarding luminal and vessel wall morphology before and after intervention.

DIAGNOSTIC USES

Although contrast angiography remains the gold standard for determining patency and continuity of blood vessels, several other imaging technologies have assumed increasingly important roles in the diagnosis of vascular disease. Noninvasive methods, including computerized tomography, magnetic resonance imaging, and duplex ultrasound, supplement the information provided by more invasive procedures such as angiography, angioscopy, and ILUS. The combined information obtained by these techniques allows examination of vascular pathology and the effects of intervention in unique and exciting ways.

Arterial Dissection

ILUS provides valuable information in the investigation of arterial wall dissections by determining the size, location, and extent of the flap and false lumen[7] (Fig 5). Because ILUS is a dynamic, real-time imaging modality, the movement of arterial dissection flaps with the systolic pulse wave can be seen. The precise location and orientation of the flap is important, since it determines the need for treatment by repair, excision, and grafting or vascular stenting. 3D ILUS is especially useful in this role, since major arterial dissection commonly results in a spiral or complex-shaped false lumen that is difficult to appreciate in three dimensions using alternative imaging methods. 3D image reconstruction of aortic dissections allows identification of the dissection entry site, extent of the flap, and relation of the false lumen to major visceral branches. Accurate assessment of these features is vital for successful experimental endoluminal stenting of aortic dissection[8] (Fig 6).

Dimensions and Morphology of Diseased Vessels

If bypass surgery remained the only method of treating peripheral vascular disease, there would be little practical value in examining the diseased

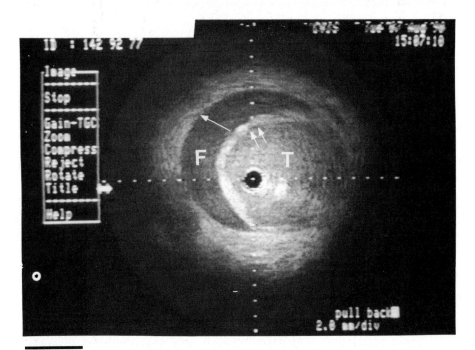

FIGURE 5.

Intraluminal ultrasound image of distal abdominal aorta in a patient with acute aortic dissection. T = true lumen; F = false lumen; *single arrow* = aortic wall; *double arrow* = dissection flap. (From Cavaye DM, French WJ, White RA, et al: *J Vasc Surg* 1991; 13:510–512. Used by permission.)

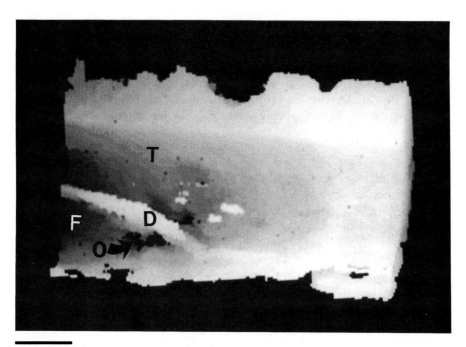

FIGURE 6.
Three-dimensional intraluminal ultrasound image of aortic dissection showing
the dissection flap *(D)*, renal artery orifice *(O)*, and false *(F)* and true *(T)* lumina.
(From Cavaye DM, Lerman RD, Kopchok GE, et al: *Am J Cardiol* 1992; 69:705–
707. Used by permission.)

portion of the vessel with any method apart from contrast angiography.
Angiography provides the anatomic data required for successful bypass
by identifying the site and extent of disease and the adequacy of inflow
and outflow vessels. Surgical intervention has continued to develop, however, and now entails a variety of options, including bypass, endarterectomy, balloon angioplasty, atherectomy, laser ablation, and intravascular
stenting. From the established to the experimental, a need now exists to
assess more accurately and objectively the diseased tissue itself, the natural history of the atherosclerotic vessel wall, the morphologic changes
produced by newer interventions, and the phenomenon of restenosis.
Studies comparing ILUS and angiography have shown that angiography
underestimates the extent of disease in vessels that contain either extensive or eccentrically located atheroma[6, 9] (Fig 7). Also, calculation of the
percent stenosis as assessed by ILUS is not the same as that determined
by angiography, since the reference vessel, which may appear free of disease angiographically, very often contains significant atheroma when examined by ILUS (Fig 8). ILUS has been used to demonstrate and localize
aortic coarctation, both experimentally and in patients who were treated
concomitantly with aortic balloon angioplasty.[10] In this study, ILUS
clearly showed the coarctation and accurately measured the adjacent normal aortic lumen for balloon sizing.

Characterization of Plaque, and Intraluminal and Intimal Lesions
In addition to providing accurate dimensional morphology, ILUS can differentiate plaque from thrombus and determine the consistency of lesions

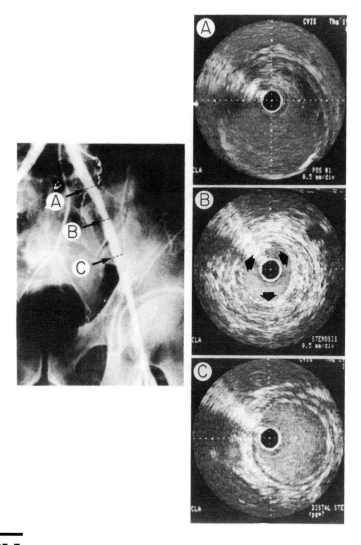

FIGURE 7.

Comparison of angiography and intraluminal ultrasound in the common and external iliac arteries. A = normal lumen; B = severe stenosis in the external iliac artery; C = normal vessel distal to the lesion. Note the three-layer appearance of this muscular artery wall in the normal segments. *Arrows* delineate a 77% cross-sectional area luminal compromise. (From Tabbara MR, White RA, Cavaye DM, et al: *J Vasc Surg* 1991; 14:496–504. Used by permission.)

and the degree of calcification present[11] (Fig 9). This information is important in determining the most suitable approach to revascularization using endovascular methods. The presence of extensive calcium within the vessel wall is a predictor of more severe medial dissection following balloon angioplasty than is its presence in vessels with minimal calcified atheroma.[12] The spatial distribution of atheroma within the vessel and the eccentricity of the lumen in relation to the vessel boundary are seen easily using ILUS, especially with longitudinal computerized reconstruction (Fig 10). Both angioscopy and ILUS are more sensitive than uniplanar angiography in identifying intimal flaps and intraluminal thrombus,

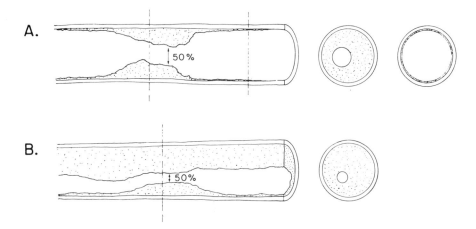

FIGURE 8.

Luminal cross-sectional depictions of arterial lesions viewed along the length *(left)* and at cross-sections made at 90 degrees to the vessel axis *(right)*. In short segmental lesions **(A)**, angiographic estimation of luminal compromise is accurate only if the adjacent normal-appearing vessel has minimal plaque. In a severely diseased vessel **(B)**, an angiographically determined 50% stenosis underestimates the volume of plaque significantly. (From Cavaye DM, White RA: *Intravascular Ultrasound Imaging.* New York, Raven Press, 1992. Used by permission.)

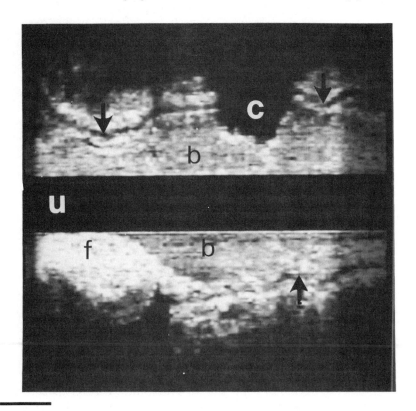

FIGURE 9.

Longitudinal gray-scale intraluminal ultrasound reconstruction of atheromatous iliac artery. Ultrasound catheter *(u)* is surrounded by blood *(b)*, with the media visible as a hypoechoic *(arrows)* layer between the hyperechoic intima and adventitia. Fibrous plaque *(f)* appears as a bright hyperechoic lesion and calcified plaque *(c)* produces a dense acoustic shadow beyond the lesion. (From Cavaye DM, Tabbara M, Kopchok G, et al: *J Vasc Surg* 1992; 16:509–519. Used by permission.)

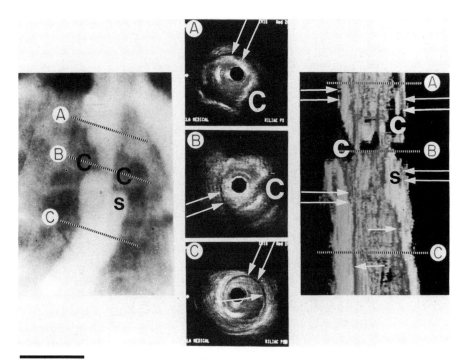

FIGURE 10.

Angiogram *(left)*, 2D intraluminal ultrasound *(center)*, and three-dimensional intraluminal ultrasound *(right)* of an atherosclerotic common iliac artery. Labels *A*, *B*, and *C* correspond to the same sites on the angiogram and three-dimensional ultrasound reconstruction. In the ultrasound images, *double arrows* mark the hypoechoic media and *single arrows* mark the luminal surface in the relatively normal arterial segment. Calcified areas *(C)* in the lesion are differentiated from soft plaque *(S)* by attenuation of the image beyond calcification. (From Cavaye DM, White RA: *J Vasc Surg* 1992; 15:1080–1081. Used by permission.)

and endovascular management of these defects has been shown to be effective in most cases.[13, 14] ILUS has been reported as a useful preoperative imaging technique for evaluating the proximal extension of intracaval renal tumor and the degree of tumor adherence within the vena cava.[10]

THERAPEUTIC USES

Therapeutic applications are developing rapidly, with ILUS being used as both a guidance modality for endovascular devices and for immediate postprocedural assessment of the effects of intervention. Improvements in ultrasound catheter resolution and the introduction of 3D image reconstruction have provided a more complete understanding of the morphology of endovascular recanalization and current failure mechanisms.

Balloon Angioplasty

Various mechanisms have been proposed to explain the arterial dilatation produced by balloon angioplasty, including compression and redistribution of plaque,[15] and stretching or dissection of the media and plaque rupture.[16] Despite postmortem histologic studies, experimentally controlled animal models, and angiographically based clinical observations,

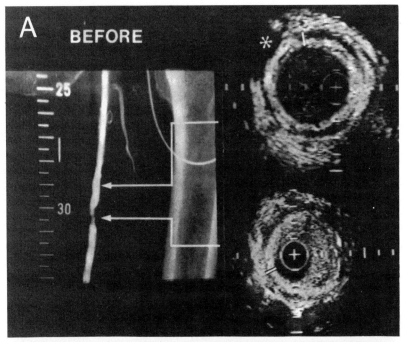

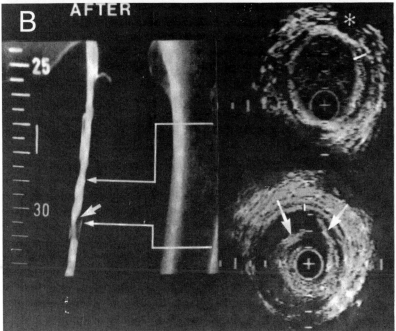

FIGURE 11.

Angiograms and intraluminal ultrasound (ILUS) images of superficial femoral artery stenosis before **(A)** and after **(B)** balloon angioplasty. ILUS images of the artery proximal to the lesion *(upper)* and at the stenosis *(lower)* are shown. Note the change in appearance of the ILUS images at the stenosis following angioplasty, with an increased area bounded by the media (wall stretching) and dissection, plaque rupture, and creation of intraluminal flaps *(arrows)*. (From The SHK, Gussenhoven EJ, Zhong Y, et al: *Circulation* 1992; 86:483–493. Used by permission.)

consensus on the precise contribution of each mechanism has not been reached. ILUS allows accurate measurement of cross-sectional luminal dimensions and illustrates the morphologic changes produced by balloon dilatation. Studies using ILUS imaging in peripheral vessels have shown that luminal enlargement by balloon dilatation is achieved primarily by overstretching the arterial wall, with the lesion volume remaining practically unchanged. Overstretching almost always is accompanied by medial dissection and plaque rupture, and occasionally by internal elastic lamina rupture[17] (Fig 11). In addition to elucidating the morphologic changes of balloon angioplasty, ILUS provides a technique for accurately measuring the luminal dimensions associated with dilatation, especially cross-sectional area and plaque volume. An important innovation that incorporates an ILUS transducer into an angioplasty balloon (Balloon Ultrasound Imaging Catheter, Boston Scientific, Watertown, Mass) allows visualization of the balloon dilatation process in real time, providing quantitative and qualitative analyses of lumen-plaque-wall alterations immediately preceding, during, and immediately after percutaneous transluminal angioplasty.[18] This device has been especially valuable in determining the degree to which vessel recoil contributes to a poor angioplasty result, and provides a reliable guide to the need for further intervention, such as repeat dilatation using a larger balloon or use of an intravascular stent. Recent studies have indicated that balloon size selection for angioplasty often is underestimated using angiography, and that ILUS provides a more accurate method for optimizing balloon-to-vessel size matching.[19, 20]

Intravascular Stents

Intravascular stents have been investigated for over 2 decades as a method to hold the vessel open mechanically and force intimal flaps and medial

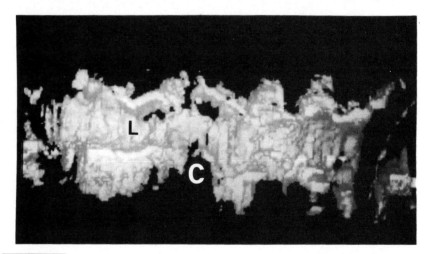

FIGURE 12.

Three-dimensional intraluminal ultrasound image of iliac artery after laser angioplasty. The vessel lumen is irregular with evidence of intimal debris, and calcified plaque *(C)* is protruding into the lumen *(L)* with acoustic shadowing behind it. (From Cavaye DM, Diethrich EB, Lass TA: *Int Angiol*, in press. Used by permission.)

dissections against the vessel wall. Recent studies suggest that the use of an intravascular stent in specific circumstances may reduce the complications of endovascular therapy related to major dissection, vessel recoil, and spasm.[21] The two important issues that are critical to the successful use of intravascular stents, whether they are used in conjunction with laser energy ablation, mechanical atherectomy, or balloon angioplasty, are (1) accurate assessment of the result of the primary intervention (i.e., is a

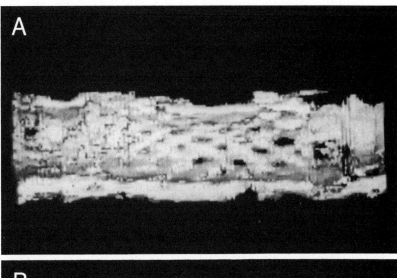

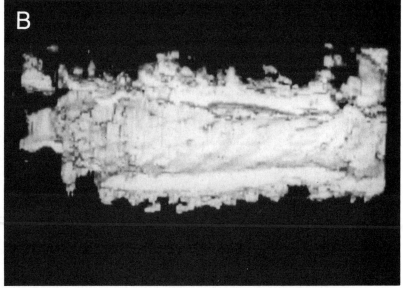

FIGURE 13.

A, three-dimensional intraluminal ultrasound image of the iliac artery shown in Figure 12, following initial stent deployment. The plaque is displaced from the lumen and the intimal surface appears smoother. A "lattice" pattern of stent struts is seen, suggesting incomplete expansion. **B,** following further balloon expansion, the stent is deployed fully, with all struts abutting the vessel wall, and a smooth luminal contour is seen. (From Cavaye DM, Diethrich EB, Lass TA: *Int Angiol,* in press. Used by permission.)

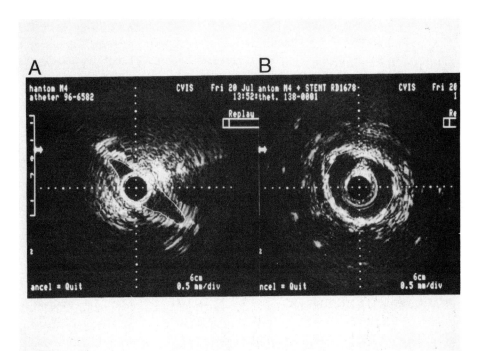

FIGURE 14.

Intraluminal images **(A)** before and **(B)** after insertion of a 5.0-mm-diameter self-expanding stent into a human superficial femoral artery in vitro. Dramatic change in luminal shape is observed, resulting in an increase in cross-sectional luminal area from 7.9 mm² to 16.7 mm². (From Cavaye DM, Tabbara M, Kopchok G, et al: *Ann Vasc Surg* 1991; 5:241–246. Used by permission.)

stent required?), and (2) stent selection and confirmation of deployment. In this regard, angiography has been shown to underestimate the degree of residual stenosis following atherectomy in up to 80% of patients, and had been unable to identify incomplete deployment in up to 20% of cases in which a stent was used.[22] ILUS imaging provides a technique with which to assess accurately the immediate results of intervention and to determine the need for an intravascular stent based on parameters such as degree of recoil, presence of flaps and dissections, and size of the residual lumen (Fig 12). By viewing both the 2D and 3D images simultaneously, correct stent and balloon size can be achieved, and the stent can be positioned accurately in relation to vessel bifurcations or major branches. Furthermore, incomplete stent deployment, as evidenced by the stent struts not fully apposing the vessel wall (appearing as a "lattice" pattern on the 3D image), can be identified and further expansion performed (Fig 13). The dimensional accuracy of standard 2D ILUS imaging of stented vessels has been confirmed, but has not been established in 3D computerized image reconstructions[11, 23] (Fig 14).

A recent experimental application of ILUS has been reported in the management of acute aortic dissection. Treatment of this disease remains controversial, with high overall mortality persisting despite advances in both operative and nonoperative management. ILUS has been used successfully in detecting experimental aortic dissections in canines and for determining the effectiveness of intravascular stenting as primary treatment alone.[8] This combination of ILUS and intravascular stents provides an exciting new experimental method for percutaneous diagnosis and treatment of acute aortic dissection, and challenges the clinician treating this disease to reexamine the controversy of surgical vs. medical therapy and to consider a possible third alternative.

Laser Angioplasty and Mechanical Atherectomy

ILUS is being investigated as a method to study the mechanism of action and results of mechanical atherectomy and laser angioplasty catheters. For each type of device, the combination of ILUS guidance and lesion assessment capabilities with the therapeutic device may improve the results of intervention in various lesions and vessels. The combination of ILUS and lasers is particularly appealing for the manufacture of cost-effective, miniaturized, precise ablation devices, since the fiberoptic and microchip components can be integrated into a single low-profile catheter. Initial investigations have demonstrated that ILUS-guided laser recanalization of experimental arterial occlusions can be achieved by concentric enlargement of the initial single-fiber channel using a larger-diameter multifiber laser catheter[24] (Fig 15). Although this type of ILUS guidance is applicable to any form of endovascular recanalization technique, including lasers and rotational or directional atherectomy, the resultant combined ILUS-therapeutic device must meet the prerequisite of cost-effective miniaturization. Imaging of arterial lesions and interventions using 3D ILUS enhances the practicality of the guided ablation concept by

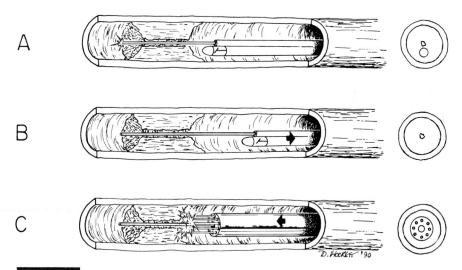

FIGURE 15.

Schematic of intraluminal ultrasound–guided laser recanalization of an experimental arterial occlusion. **A,** laser fiberoptic centered in the vessel lumen by coaxial alignment with the ultrasound catheter tip, followed by advancement of the fiber through the occlusion. **B,** withdrawal of the ultrasound catheter, leaving the laser fiberoptic positioned in the lesion. **C,** passage of the multifiber laser catheter over the single fiberoptic to enlarge the vessel lumen concentrically. (From White RA, Kopchok GE, Tabbara MR, et al: *Lasers Surg Med* 1992; 12:239–245. Used by permission.)

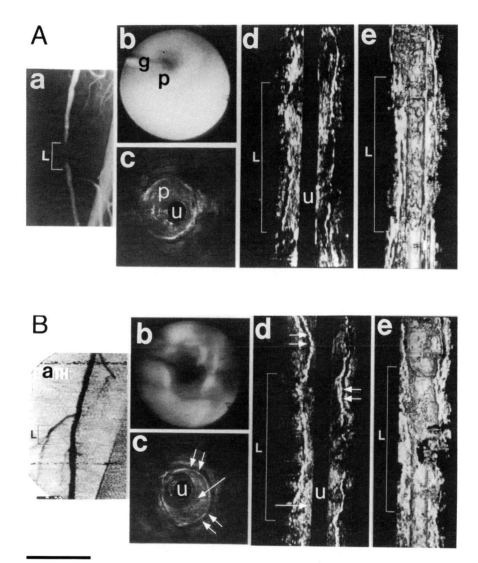

FIGURE 16.

Comparison of angiography (a), angioscopy (b), and intraluminal ultrasound cross-sectional (c), longitudinal (d), and three-dimensional reconstructions (e) before **(A)** and after **(B)** recanalization of a superficial femoral artery localized occlusion. Before the intervention, the lesion completely fills the lumen, with plaque (p) abutting the guidewire (g) on the angioscopic image. After rotational atherectomy, the angiogram of the lesion suggests that the plaque was removed completely when compared to the appearance of the adjacent "normal" artery. Although angioscopy shows a significantly larger lumen, intraluminal ultrasound demonstrates that the majority of the area bounded by the media (double arrows) is occupied by residual plaque (single arrows) and occupies more than 60% of the luminal volume of the vessel in three dimensions. L= lesion; u = intraluminal ultrasound catheter. (From Cavaye DM, White RA: Intravascular Ultrasound Imaging. New York, Raven Press, 1992, pp 88–89. Used by permission.)

providing an easily interpretable reconstruction of the vessel and recanalization. By assimilating hundreds of cross-sectional ILUS images into a single-vessel reconstruction that displays the spatial arrangement of eccentrically positioned or variable-consistency plaque, 3D ILUS provides a unique method for viewing endovascular recanalization procedures.

Recurrent stenosis or occlusion of vascular segments treated with these ablative devices remains a major obstacle to further development of endovascular treatment of symptomatic atherosclerosis. The approach to the problem of restenosis must be well controlled, with the individual roles of contributing factors such as thrombosis, inadequate lesion removal, smooth muscle cell proliferation and migration, and progression of atherosclerosis being examined in isolation. If the combined effects of these factors are considered generically to be "restenosis," efforts to control a single cause in isolation (e.g., smooth muscle cell hyperplasia) may lead to spurious conclusions because of the unrecognized roles of the other modes of postangioplasty stenosis. In most cases, failures currently attributed to smooth muscle cell hyperplasia are caused by inadequate removal of atherosclerotic lesions or by thrombosis and reorganization of residual debris. The reported high recurrence rates of almost all interventional methods are caused by a combination of poor lesion debulking and trauma to the vessel wall, which stimulates a proliferative reaction that is pathophysiologically similar to the normal process of wound healing within the vessel.

Contributing to this potential confusion is the inadequacy of angiography to provide accurate control data before and after intervention (Fig 16). ILUS may play a pivotal role in the investigation of angioplasty restenosis by defining the types and spatial distribution of disease and providing precise control cross-sectional dimensions of the vessel before and after intervention.

CURRENT LIMITATIONS AND FUTURE DIRECTIONS

ILUS imaging currently is limited by the relatively high cost of disposable catheters and by its invasive nature. Its diagnostic applications will be relevant only in cases in which concomitant invasive diagnostic studies are performed (e.g., peripheral angiography or cardiac catheterization) or as a guidance component of a therapeutic device (e.g., stent deployment or angioplasty). Major priorities in the ongoing development of ILUS are the need for further miniaturization and cost-effective manufacturing. Current devices are relatively expensive and, if the technique is to be of clinical benefit as a component of a disposable catheter system for diagnostic or therapeutic intervention, the price of individual units must be justified by the benefits of ILUS imaging.

Although it has been shown that 2D cross-sectional ILUS and computerized longitudinal reconstructions provide accurate luminal and transmural measurements, the dimensional accuracy of currently available 3D imaging has not been established. By viewing all three image formats simultaneously on a screen, however, the location of the 2D image site along the length of the 3D image can be identified using a linear cursor, and dimensions of a site on the 3D image can be estimated. A continuing problem associated with many 3D imaging techniques is the near-field effect of the ultrasound imaging catheters at frequencies of 20 to 30 MHz, resulting in bright imaging of the blood immediately surrounding the catheter. As the 3D imaging software has improved, it has allowed manipulation of the image data to reduce the blood artifact, but this problem still remains in some images because of the inherent features of the imaging catheter.

Future angioplasty guidance devices may combine the benefits of angioscopy and intravascular ultrasound in a single, disposable delivery system suitable for incorporation into any mechanical or laser-based ablation device. Angioscopy would allow visual inspection of the lumen, with ultrasound determining the vessel wall characteristics and dimensions. An added benefit of this type of guidance device would be the ability to select an appropriate ablation method for particular plaque types or volumes. ILUS imaging also provides an exciting opportunity for vascular research, including investigation of blood vessel compliance, dynamic changes in the vascular wall caused by disease or pharmacologic intervention, and the natural history of atherosclerosis.

REFERENCES

1. Lockwood GR, Ryan LK, Foster FS: High frequency intravascular ultrasound imaging, in Cavaye DM, White RA (eds): *A Text and Atlas of Arterial Imaging*. London, Chapman & Hall, 1992, pp 135–137.
2. Raya SP, Udupa JK, Barrett WA: A PC-based 3D imaging system: Algorithms, software and hardware considerations. *Comput Med Imaging Graph* 1990; 14:353–370.
3. Gussenhoven WJ, Essed CE, Frietman P, et al: Intravascular echographic assessment of vessel wall characteristics: A correlation with histology. *Int J Card Imaging* 1989; 4:105–116.
4. Kopchok GE, White RA, Guthrie C, et al: Intraluminal vascular ultrasound: Preliminary report of dimensional and morphologic accuracy. *Ann Vasc Surg* 1990; 4:291–296.
5. Mallery JA, Tobis JM, Griffith J, et al: Assessment of normal and atherosclerotic arterial wall thickness with an intravascular ultrasound imaging catheter. *Am Heart J* 1990; 119:1392–1400.
6. Tabbara MR, White RA, Cavaye DM, et al: In-vivo human comparison of intravascular ultrasound and angiography. *J Vasc Surg* 1991; 14:496–504.
7. Cavaye DM, French WJ, White RA, et al: Intravascular ultrasound assessment of an acute dissecting aortic aneurysm: A case report. *J Vasc Surg* 1991; 13:510–512.
8. Cavaye DM, Lerman RD, Kopchok GE, et al: Usefulness of intravascular ultrasound imaging for detecting experimentally induced aortic dissection in dogs and for determining the effectiveness of endoluminal stenting. *Am J Cardiol* 1992; 69:705–707.
9. Tobis JM, Mahon D, Lehmann K, et al: The sensitivity of ultrasound imaging compared with angiography for diagnosing coronary atherosclerosis (abstract). *Circulation* 1990; 82(suppl III):439.
10. Barone GW, Kahn MB, Cook JM, et al: Recurrent intracaval renal cell carcinoma: The role of intravascular ultrasonography. *J Vasc Surg* 1991; 13:506–509.
11. Cavaye DM, White RA, Kopchok GE, et al: Three dimensional intravascular

ultrasound imaging of normal and diseased, canine and human arteries. *J Vasc Surg* 1992; 16:509–519.

12. Fitzgerald PJ, Ports TA, Yock PG: Contribution of localized calcium deposits to dissection after angioplasty: An observational study using intravascular ultrasound. *Circulation* 1992; 86:64–70.

13. Neville RF, Yasuhara H, Watanabe BI, et al: Endovascular management of arterial intimal defects: An experimental comparison by arteriography, angioscopy and intravascular ultrasonography. *J Vasc Surg* 1991; 13:496–502.

14. White GH, White RA, Kopchok GE, et al: Endoscopic intravascular surgery removes intraluminal flaps, dissections and thrombus. *J Vasc Surg* 1990; 11:280–288.

15. Dotter CT, Judkins MP: Transluminal treatment of atherosclerotic obstruction: Description of a new technique and a preliminary report of its application. *Circulation* 1964; 30:654–670.

16. Lyon RT, Zarins CK, Lu CT, et al: Vessel, plaque and lumen morphology after transluminal balloon angioplasty: Quantitative study in distended human arteries. *Arteriosclerosis* 1987; 7:306–314.

17. The SHK, Gussenhoven EJ, Zhong Y, et al: Effect of balloon angioplasty on femoral artery evaluated with intravascular ultrasound imaging. *Circulation* 1992; 86:483–493.

18. Isner JM, Rosenfield K, Losordo DW, et al: Combination balloon-ultrasound imaging catheter for percutaneous transluminal angioplasty. *Circulation* 1991; 84:739–754.

19. Cacchione J, Nair R, Hodson J: Intracoronary ultrasound: Better than conventional methods for determining optimal PTCA balloon size (abstract). *J Am Coll Cardiol* 1991; 17:112A.

20. Rothman A, Ricou F, Weintraub RG, et al: Intraluminal ultrasound imaging through a balloon dilation catheter in an animal model of coarctation of the aorta. *Circulation* 1992; 85:2291–2295.

21. Palmaz JC, Garcia OJ, Schatz RA, et al: Placement of balloon expandable intraluminal stents in iliac arteries: First 171 procedures. *Radiology* 1990; 174:969–975.

22. Katzen BT, Benenati JF, Becker GJ, et al: Role of intravascular ultrasound in peripheral atherectomy and stent deployment (abstract). *Circulation* 1991; 84(suppl II):2152.

23. Cavaye DM, Tabbara MR, Kopchok GE, et al: Intraluminal ultrasound assessment of vascular stent deployment. *Ann Vasc Surg* 1991; 5:230–236.

24. White RA, Kopchok GE, Tabbara MR, et al: Intravascular ultrasound guided holmium:YAG laser recanalization of occluded arteries. *Lasers Surg Med* 1992; 12:239–245.

The Role of Angioscopy in Infrainguinal Arterial Reconstructions

WILLIAM H. PEARCE, M.D.

KEVIN D. NOLAN, M.D., M.P.H.

JAMES S.T. YAO, M.D., PH.D.

T he role of angioscopy in lower extremity bypass procedures is in a state of evolution. High-resolution, small-diameter angioscopes with microchip cameras, video monitoring, and dedicated irrigating systems permit clear visualization of the lumina of arteries and veins. As with any new technology, an initial wave of enthusiasm has accompanied the application of angioscopy to a wide variety of vascular procedures. However, the real value of angioscopy will be determined only with generalized clinical experience and randomized prospective trials. Since angioscopy provides a visual image, it has been assumed that it must offer some advantage over the "blind" techniques that frequently are used during valve lysis for in situ vein bypasses and the passage of Fogarty catheters for thromboembolectomies. Angioscopy also may prove to be more sensitive than completion of arteriography in detecting technical errors following lower extremity bypasses. Although these arguments may have merit, there are few data to support the routine use of angioscopy during infrainguinal reconstruction. This chapter will review the development of both the equipment and its use during in situ vein bypass and thromboembolectomy, as well as its role in the detection of technical defects during infrainguinal bypass.

HISTORY

Prior to the development of cardiopulmonary bypass, attempts to perform endoscopy of the cardiovascular system were limited to the heart. Rigid endoscopes with lens systems were used to visualize intracardiac pathology, but proved too large for use in peripheral vessels. In 1966, Greenstone and colleagues used a rigid choledochoscope to view the lumina of larger arteries in dogs and human cadavers.[1] In 1974, Vollmar and Storz first reported on angioscopy in clinical practice using a flexible choledochoscope.[2] Further clinical experience was reported by Crispin and Van Baarle in 1973[3] and then by Towne and Bernhard in 1977.[4] The authors concurred that angioscopy was a safe technique and a potential alterna-

Advances in Vascular Surgery, vol. 1.
©1993, Mosby–Year Book, Inc.

tive to completion arteriography. Recent investigators using modern angioscopes and video equipment have confirmed these earlier experiences. These reports offer few objective data, however, and fail to define precise clinical advantages provided by routine angioscopy.[5-8]

With the development of endovascular surgical techniques (laser and atherectomy), a heightened demand for angioscopy was generated. Angioscopy allowed the surgeon to guide such instruments under direct vision and, theoretically, limit laser ablation or atherectomy to the diseased arterial segment.[9] Endovascular surgery using angioscopy also was favored as an adjunct to performing the in situ bypass.[10-12] The technical success or failure of one of these procedures could be viewed directly with the angioscope. Unfortunately, clinical results using angioscopy to perform endovascular surgery have been only anecdotal.

Nevertheless, there appears to be a definite advantage of angioscopy over completion arteriography in detecting technical errors.[6,12-14] Anastomotic narrowing, intimal flaps, and retained uncut valve leaflets not apparent on completion arteriography are seen readily with the angioscope. Although magnification by the angioscope allows accurate identification of intraluminal morphology, the significance of these lesions remains obscure in the absence of data regarding the natural history. Small fragments of intima frequently are observed floating in the lumen without obstruction, and it is unclear whether they should be removed. Only with time and clinical experience is it possible that clinically useful decisions may be made on the basis of angioscopic findings.

EQUIPMENT

Angioscopes, cameras, monitors, and other video components are readily available from several different sources. Many different sizes of angioscopes are available, but only three are used in the operating rooms at Northwestern University: a 1.4-mm solid nonsteerable scope without an irrigating channel, a 2.2-mm steerable solid scope that allows a deflection of 120 degrees without an irrigation channel, and a 2.8-mm nonsteerable scope with a 1-mm irrigation channel. A 300-W xenon light source is used. The angioscope is coupled with a camera, video monitor, and .5-in. videocassette recorder. Still photography may be obtained with special additional equipment.

An important piece of equipment is a dedicated system for irrigation capable of clearing the lumen of blood. Our system provides for high and low flow rates with a continuous digital readout of the volume of fluid infused, which is a particularly helpful feature that minimizes inadvertent fluid overload. This pump is volume-driven, however, and excessive pressure may develop in closed vascular segments, producing deleterious overdistention and damage to the conduit. Careful attention must be paid to both volume and infusion pressure.

ANGIOSCOPY-ASSISTED IN SITU BYPASS

For the first time since the original description of the in situ bypass by Hall in 1962, angioscopy permits visualization of venous valvulotomy.[15]

Valve incision performed during an in situ bypass relies upon retrograde pressure (either arterial or from an irrigation catheter) to close the valve mechanism. A valvulotome is inserted and the venous leaflet is incised blindly. The vein wall may be injured at any point, but injury is particularly likely when the leaflet is adjacent to a small side branch. The use of angioscopy to monitor valvulotomy was introduced by Fleisher and associates in 1986.[10] Damage to the venous conduit could be avoided and arteriovenous fistulas could be identified using the angioscope. In this preliminary report, angioscopy did not prolong the operative procedure and was not associated with fluid overload. Later reports by Matsumoto[11] and Mehigan[12] and their colleagues confirmed the utility of angioscopy in performing in situ bypass and led to their recommendation that the angioscope be used for the preparation of translocated vein segments. Residual intact valve leaflets and persistent arteriovenous fistulas were avoided using this method.

It is difficult to advocate the routine use of angioscopy for the experienced surgeon who has had excellent results with other techniques. However, the greatest benefit of angioscopy is the ability to confirm visually complete valve lysis. With other techniques, incomplete valvulotomy and unrecognized vein wall trauma may occur. In a prospective study of 250 in situ bypass procedures, Bandyk and colleagues identified 21 graft problems with surveillance duplex scanning that were either retained valve leaflets, residual arteriovenous fistulas, or anastomotic stenoses.[16] Miller and coworkers performed routine angioscopy following infrainguinal bypass and found a 17% incidence of retained valve leaflets and a 60% incidence of residual arteriovenous fistulas.[5] These partially torn valves may create turbulent blood flow and become the site of vein graft stenosis. In our own experience, angioscopy detected mid-vein graft abnormalities in only 4% of patients, all of which were unrelated to incomplete valvulotomy; the lesions identified occurred in sclerotic vein segments.[14] Recently, there has been enthusiasm to perform angioscopy to identify vein abnormalities prior to all vein bypass procedures. Since the incidence of undetected vein abnormalities in our experience is so low (4%), prebypass angioscopy is not carried out routinely. Rather, these abnormalities are found subsequently with completion angioscopy and are corrected then. Similar results have been noted by Mehigan and Olcott, who found only one retained functional valve leaflet and three patent side branches in 55 patients.[12]

An additional benefit of angioscopy is that the operation may be performed without the long leg incision required for exposure of the full length of the vein. A high wound complication rate has been reported in association with these long incisions.[17] Since it is possible to identify major side branches with the angioscope, only small cutdowns are required for their ligation. The below-the-knee incision for tibial artery bypasses still is required, however, and it is precisely in this area that the majority of wound problems occur.

Despite these potential advantages, the angioscope theoretically may produce more endothelial cell damage than do other methods. A relatively large angioscope with other endovascular instruments and forceful irrigation may denude long arterial segments. Therefore, it is critically important to use the smallest angioscope possible and to avoid high distending pressures. In a small-diameter vein, angioscopy should be avoided altogether. Fluid overload with high-flow irrigation systems is always a possibility. In our experience and that of others, the amount of fluid usually infused ranges between 500 and 1,500 mL. Much of this is lost through the open distal vein, and infusions in excess of 2,000 cc are rare for in situ bypass.

As with other new technologies, the value of the angioscope in performing the in situ bypass must be reviewed critically. There have been no long-term, prospective, randomized studies that define a clear benefit for angioscopy in this procedure. However, preliminary reports suggest that potential benefits may derive from visually confirmed valve lysis and avoidance of retained arteriovenous fistulas.

TECHNIQUE

Incision of the venous valves with the aid of the angioscope is performed following routine exposure of the saphenous vein, femoral vessels, and recipient popliteal/tibial vessels. After the proximal venous valves are incised under direct vision, the angioscope and irrigating system are introduced either through the transected end of the saphenous vein or through large proximal side branches.

A special flexible valvulotome, 100 cm long and equipped with a detachable cutting blade (2.5 mm) is passed from below using the blunt tip. The cutting blade then is secured for valve incision. The angioscope and irrigating system are introduced through the proximal open end of the saphenous vein, which is encircled with a vessel loop. Occasionally, it is difficult to maintain a water seal with the vessel loop alone and additional digital pressure may be required. An alternative method is to complete the proximal anastomosis while preserving several large side branches. One branch provides access for the irrigation system and the second is used for the angioscope. Once the angioscope is inserted, the vein is distended gently. With continued gentle irrigation, blood entering from the tributaries is removed and the valve leaflets and cutting instruments can be seen (Fig 1). The cutting instrument is placed at the leading edge of the closed valve and the valve leaflet is incised. Occasionally, the valve mechanism is adjacent to a side branch, allowing the cutting edge of the valvulotome to lodge inadvertently in the orifice of the tributary. With direct visualization provided by the angioscope, it is possible to redirect the valvulotome for accurate valve incision. Once both valve leaflets have been cut, the valve mechanism is irrigated to confirm unobstructed flow.

Large venous tributaries are identified either by passing the angioscope into their lumina or by placing the cutting instrument into their orifices. Transillumination from the light of the angioscope identifies the segment for dissection. This technique is particularly useful when a long skin incision is not used to expose the vein. Instead, several small skin incisions are made over the transilluminated skin and subcutaneous tissue to ligate arteriovenous fistulas.

The angioscope and valvulotome are passed down the vein, sequentially disrupting each valve mechanism encountered. Once all of the val-

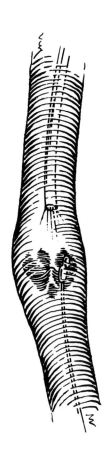

FIGURE 1.

Venous valvulotomy with angioscopy. The angioscope is proximal to the venous valve and valvulotome.

vulotomies have been performed, the angioscope is withdrawn, checking each valve for function. The distal anastomosis then is completed in a standard fashion.

ANGIOSCOPICALLY ASSISTED THROMBOEMBOLECTOMY

The treatment of lower extremity arterial emboli has not changed significantly since the introduction of the Fogarty catheter in 1963. In combination with systemic heparinization, the Fogarty catheter has greatly increased rates of initial limb salvage from 70% to 99%.[18] Thromboembolectomy using the Fogarty catheter is a blind procedure. The catheter is placed in the distal arterial system and is withdrawn using a subjective estimation of arterial drag to remove intraluminal material effectively while minimizing endothelial damage. It frequently is difficult to cannulate each of the tibial vessels selectively. As a result, some combination of J wires, fluoroscopy, and mechanical bending of the catheter tip is used to guide the catheter into each of the tibial vessels.[17, 19] On occasion, it becomes necessary to cut down upon the infrapopliteal vessels directly to guide the catheter manually into appropriate distal vessels. Less frequently, arteriotomy is required for passage of the catheter into each tib-

ial vessel and adjunctive patch angioplasty may become necessary for closure.

Intraoperative arteriography is performed to define runoff and to
search for residual thrombi. Commonly, distal thrombi and debris remain
after an "adequate" blind thromboembolectomy.[6, 20, 21] It is unclear, however, whether total extraction of residual thrombus enhances limb salvage
beyond that achieved with the intrinsic fibrinolytic system.

Angioscopy offers the ability to direct the Fogarty catheter into the
tibial vessels, obviating the necessity for fluoroscopy or distal popliteal
artery exposure. Under direct vision, the Fogarty catheter is guided into
the appropriate tibial vessel and intraluminal material is extracted. Since
angioscopy does not provide information regarding the status of the distal runoff vessels, intraoperative arteriography remains essential to define
distal tibial and pedal anatomy. Furthermore, angioscopy-assisted thromboembolectomy may diminish catheter-related injuries by allowing direct
visualization of thromboembolectomy while the procedure is being performed.[21] In theory, under direct vision, distention of the balloon catheter is limited to an amount just sufficient to remove the thrombus. To date,
few data are available to confirm this hypothesis. In addition, large-bore
angioscopes used coaxially with Fogarty catheters may produce significant intimal damage and the same adverse effects as occur with an over-
distended balloon catheter.

Angioscopy is useful in thromboembolectomy of prosthetic grafts,
which are devoid of an intimal lining and, therefore, are vulnerable in a
normal vessel. The pseudointima may be disrupted by the Fogarty catheter, however, producing free-floating debris. Removal of this debris is
essential to ensure adequate prograde flow and to prevent distal embolization.[22] Angioscopy is valuable in identifying such midgraft debris and
for inspecting the proximal and distal anastomoses. Mechanical graft
kinking may be identified also. Unfortunately, data again are insufficient
to suggest whether angioscopy-assisted thromboembolectomy offers any
advantage over current "blind" methods.

In preliminary studies, angioscopy as an adjunctive technique seems
to improve limb salvage, yet its precise role in the management of patients with acute arterial ischemia has yet to be defined. Larger series are
needed to assess adequately the impact of angioscopy-assisted thromboembolectomy. Although residual debris, intimal flaps, and adherent
thrombi are found routinely following thromboembolectomy, the natural
history of such lesions remains largely unknown.

TECHNIQUE

The basic surgical technique employed for lower extremity angioscopy-
assisted thromboembolectomy does not differ from the standard procedure, nor do indications for operation or the need for preoperative arteriography. The common femoral artery is opened transversely and a
Fogarty catheter is passed for the retrieval of distal emboli and debris.
The angioscope then is inserted through the transverse arteriotomy along
with an irrigating catheter. Using pump-driven perfusion with volume
monitored carefully by the anesthetist and the operating surgeon, the distal arterial circulation is cleared of blood. The entire length of the super-

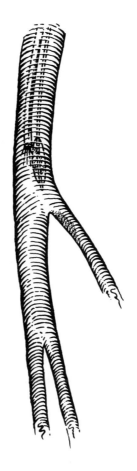

FIGURE 2.

Under direct vision, the embolectomy catheter is directed into the appropriate tibial vessel.

ficial femoral and popliteal arteries is inspected. Since the tibial-peroneal trunk and peroneal arteries are the most direct route followed by the Fogarty catheter, particularly careful inspection is made of the orifices of the posterior and anterior arteries. If embolic debris remains, the angioscope is left in a viewing position and the Fogarty catheter is guided under direct vision into the obstructed lumen (Fig 2). A gentle curve in the distal portion of the Fogarty catheter is useful for guidance. The angioscope and Fogarty catheter are removed simultaneously. In some instances, biopsy forceps or brushes have been used to dislodge adherent intraluminal thrombus. Since it appears that the brush technique is associated with significant intimal injury, we have not selected this approach and have used repeated irrigations and catheter passages in an attempt to remove residual adherent thrombi. With the recent addition of intraoperative thrombolytic therapy, angioscopy allows for objective appraisal of the efficacy of this mode of therapy. With the complete removal of any visual thrombus, the arteriotomy is closed and an intraoperative completion arteriogram is performed.

When it is necessary to perform a proximal iliac embolectomy, proximal occlusion can be obtained by inserting a balloon catheter in the aorta and withdrawing it to a position at the takeoff of the iliac vessels. If there is no significant back-bleeding from the hypogastric vessels, it is possible to examine the lumen of the external iliac and common iliac vessels. In selected cases, we have found occlusive disease in the iliac artery that was responsible for the initiation of thrombus with distal embolus.

Following graft thromboembolectomy, completion angioscopy is performed to ensure complete removal of intraluminal thrombus and loosened pseudointima. When the graft is exposed distally, a Fogarty catheter is used for proximal control. In prosthetic grafts, a large angioscope is used to inspect the proximal and distal anastomosis for evidence of neo-intimal hyperplasia. Flaps of pseudointima are removed with a flexible biopsy forceps if necessary and graft revision is performed as needed.

ANGIOSCOPY AS A TECHNIQUE TO DETECT TECHNICAL ERRORS

Successful arterial reconstruction of the lower extremity is dependent upon a number of factors, including adequate inflow, a suitable conduit, sufficient runoff, and meticulous surgical technique. From 14% to 49% of early graft failures following femoral distal bypass result from a technical error.[23] As a result, a number of different intraoperative techniques have been developed to detect intimal flaps, anastomotic narrowings, intraluminal thrombi, and kinking of the grafts. Completion arteriography is considered the gold standard by which other techniques are measured. Renwick and colleagues compared two similar groups of patients undergoing femoral popliteal reconstruction with and without completion arteriography.[24] Immediate reoperation was necessary in 18% of the patients who did not undergo completion arteriography, but in none of the patients who had completion studies. At 3 months, the cumulative patency rates were 74.5% in the control group and 91% in the group of patients who underwent completion arteriography. Although completion arteriography is highly specific, it is only a moderately sensitive test.[6, 23, 25] Other intraoperative methods used to detect technical errors include electromagnetic flow probes, B-mode scans, and Doppler spectral analysis. However, none of these techniques replaces completion arteriography. In addition to providing a means by which to assess operative technique, completion arteriography defines the runoff anatomy. Clear definition of runoff vessels is essential when planning strategy for potential reoperation and assessing the need for long-term anticoagulation. The completion arteriogram also has proved useful with late graft failures. Patent distal vessels may be used for subsequent reoperation. At our institution, copies of all completion arteriograms are maintained in a file within our offices.

Angioscopy offers yet another method by which to assess the quality of an infrainguinal bypass. In 112 lower extremity bypass procedures, Miller and associates reported that surgical decisions were made on the basis of angioscopy alone in 48% of the cases.[5] Angioscopic findings that prompted a change in the surgical procedure included incompletely cut venous valve leaflets and missed arteriovenous fistulas in in situ grafts. However, comparative intraoperative arteriograms were performed in only 16% of patients. In studies that have compared both techniques, angioscopy was more accurate than arteriography in detecting technical errors.[13, 14, 25] In one prospective study of 49 femorodistal bypasses, Baxter and coworkers found that completion arteriography was highly specific (95%), but not sensitive (67%), when compared with angioscopy.[14] The angioscopic findings in three grafts with normal arteriograms (false-negatives) revealed intimal flaps (2 grafts) and intraluminal thrombus (1 graft). In 10% of the procedures, angioscopy revealed technical problems that required an unanticipated alteration in the surgical procedure.

COMMENTS

Until recently, there have been no prospective randomized studies comparing routine angioscopy with standard operative methods to improve infrainguinal graft patency. At the 1992 annual meeting of the International Society for Cardiovascular Surgery in Chicago, Miller and colleagues[25] reported no statistical difference in early patency (30 days) between bypass grafts having either completion angioscopy or arteriography (n = 250). However, there was a clear trend in favor of angioscopy. Twelve grafts failed (4.8%), 4 in the angioscopy group (3.1%) and 8 in the control group (6.6%). In addition, clinically relevant decisions were made in 39 patients in the angioscopy group as compared with 7 in the angiogram group. Overall, angioscopy appeared to be more sensitive to the detection of midgraft and anastomotic problems than did arteriography, but less sensitive to lesions distal to the anastomosis. Thus, angioscopy and intraoperative arteriography are complementary in assessing both the graft and the runoff vessels.

The degree to which we must pursue the use of alternative techniques to assure that early graft failure will not occur due to technical problems is uncertain. In a review by Stept and colleagues[23] from our institution, early graft failure occurred in 62 of 849 cases (7.3%). Technical defects were found with angioscopy in only 9 patients (1%) that were not detected by arteriography. Other etiologies for early graft failure included embolization, coagulation disorders, and inadequate runoff, and the etiology could not be determined in 48% of patients. If technical defects occur in only 1% of cases, it becomes difficult to justify the routine use of completion angioscopy. Further studies are required to substantiate any long-term benefit for routine angioscopy.

REFERENCES

1. Greenstone SM, Shore JM, Heringman EC, et al: Arterial endoscopy (arterioscopy). *Arch Surg* 1966; 93:811–812.
2. Vollmar JF, Storz LW: Vascular endoscopy: Possibilities and limit of its clinical application. *Surg Clin North Am* 1974; 54:111–122.
3. Crispin HA, Van Baarle AF: Intravascular observation and surgery using the flexible fibrescope. *Lancet* 1973; 1:750–751.
4. Towne JB, Bernhard VM: Vascular endoscopy: Useful tool or interesting toy. *Surgery* 1977; 82:415–419.
5. Miller A, Campbell DR, Gibbons GW, et al: Routine intraoperative angioscopy in lower extremity revascularization. *Arch Surg* 1989; 124:604–608.

6. Van Stiegmann G, Pearce WH, Bartle EJ, et al: Flexible angioscopy seems faster and more specific than arteriography. *Arch Surg* 1987; 122:279–282.

7. Grundfest WS, Litvack F, Glick P, et al: Intraoperative decisions based on angioscopy in peripheral vascular surgery. *Circulation* 1988; 78(suppl I): 13–17.

8. Seeger JM, Abela GS: Angioscopy as an adjunct to arterial reconstructive surgery: A preliminary report. *J Vasc Surg* 1986; 4:315–320.

9. Van Stiegman G, Kahn D, Rose AG, et al: Endoscope laser endarterectomy. *Surg Gynecol Obstet* 1984; 158:529–534.

10. Fleisher HL, Tompson BW, McGowan TC, et al: Angioscopically monitored saphenous vein valvotomy. *J Vasc Surg* 1986; 4:360–364.

11. Matsumoto T, Hashizume M: Direct vision valvulotomy in in situ venous bypass. *Surg Gynecol Obstet* 1987; 165:362–364.

12. Mehigan JT, Olcott C IV: Video angioscopy as an alternative to intraoperative arteriography. *Am J Surg* 1986; 152:139–145.

13. White GH, White RA, Kopchok GE, et al: Intraoperative video angioscopy compared with arteriography during peripheral vascular operations. *J Vasc Surg* 1987; 6:488–495.

14. Baxter BT, Rizzo RJ, Flinn WR, et al: A comparative study of intraoperative angioscopy and completion arteriography following femorodistal bypass. *Arch Surg* 1990; 125:997–1002.

15. Hall KV: The great saphenous vein used in-situ as an arterial shunt after extirpation of the vein. *Surgery* 1962; 51:452.

16. Bandyk DF, Schmitt DD, Seabrook GR, et al: Monitoring functional patency of in situ saphenous vein bypasses: The impact of a surveillance protocol and elective revision. *J Vasc Surg* 1989; 9(2):286–296.

17. Schwartz ME, Harrington EB, Schanzer H: Wound complications after in-situ bypass. *J Vasc Surg* 1988; 7:802–807.

18. Dale WA: Differential management of acute peripheral arterial ischemia. *J Vasc Surg* 1984; 1:269–278.

19. Robicsek F: Dye-enhanced fluoroscopic directed catheter embolectomy. *Surgery* 1984; 95:622–624.

20. White GH, White RA, Kopchok GE, et al: Angioscopic thromboembolectomy: Preliminary observations with a recent technique. *J Vasc Surg* 1988; 7:318–325.

21. Schweitzer DL, Aguam AS, Wilder JR: Complications encountered during arterial embolectomy with the Fogarty balloon catheter. *J Vasc Surg* 1976; 76:144–156.

22. Puckett JW, Lindsay SF: Mid-graft currettage as a routine adjunct to salvage operations for thrombosed PTFE hemodialysis access grafts. *Am J Surg* 1988; 156:139–143.

23. Stept L, Flinn W, McCarthy WJ, et al: Technical defects as a cause of early graft failure after femorodistal bypass. *Arch Surg* 1987; 22:599–604.

24. Renwick S, Royle JP, Martin P, et al: Operative angiography after femoropopliteal arterial reconstruction: Its influence on early failure rate. *Br J Surg* 1968; 55:136.

25. Miller A, Marcaccio E, Tannenbaum G, et al: Comparison of angioscopy and angiography for monitoring infrainguinal bypass vein grafts: Results of a prospective randomized trial. *J Vasc Surg* 1992; 15:1078.

PART IV

Renal Artery Disease

Changing Concepts in Indications for Renal Artery Reconstruction

RICHARD H. DEAN, M.D.

Concepts of interventional management of renovascular disease have evolved continuously during the past 60 years. Following the 1934 demonstration of a renovascular cause of hypertension by Goldblatt in a dog model,[1] many patients were treated by nephrectomy on the basis of hypertension and a small kidney or intravenous pyelography. Curiously, there rarely was any interest in documenting a renal artery occlusive lesion in any of these patients. Dissatisfaction with the results of this form of treatment prompted Smith,[2] in 1956, to review 575 cases treated in this manner. He found only a 26% rate of cure of hypertension by nephrectomy using these criteria, which led him to suggest that nephrectomy should be limited to strict urologic indications. Two years previously, however, Freeman performed an aortic and bilateral renal artery thromboendarterectomy on a hypertensive patient, with resultant resolution of hypertension. This was the first cure of hypertension by renal revascularization.

DeCamp and Birchall,[4] Morris and associates,[5] and others[6, 7] soon followed with additional descriptions of relief of hypertension by renal revascularization. Concomitant with these reports, aortography began to be used widely. During the late 1950s, many centers were demonstrating renal artery stenosis in hypertensive patients by aortography and then performing either aortorenal bypass or thromboendarterectomy. Nevertheless, by 1960, it became apparent that revascularization in hypertensive individuals with renal artery stenosis was associated with reduction of blood pressure in less than 50% of them. General pessimism followed regarding the merits of operative treatment of hypertension.

As this experience pointed out, the coexistence of renal artery stenosis and hypertension does not establish a causal relationship. Many normotensive patients, especially those past the age of 50 years, have renal artery stenosis. Obviously, special studies are required to establish the functional significance of renal artery lesions. The most recent era in the history of operative treatment of renovascular hypertension began with the introduction of meaningful tests of split renal function by Howard and Conner,[8] and by Stamey and colleagues.[9] Furthermore, the work of Page and Helmes,[10] and that of others[11–13] in the identification of the renin-angiotensin system of blood pressure control added a new dimen-

Advances in Vascular Surgery, vol. 1.
©1993, Mosby–Year Book, Inc.

sion to our understanding of renovascular hypertension. With the later addition of accurate methods of measuring plasma renin activity, the physician could predict accurately which renal artery lesion was producing renovascular hypertension. Experience has shown that, if they are performed properly, positive results from split renal function studies or renal vein renin assays indicate that a good blood pressure response can be expected following successful operation in over 95% of cases.[14]

Flush aortography with selective renal arteriography in multiple projections might be considered the gold standard screening test. Similarly, split renal function studies and renal vein renin assays used to predict a favorable response to intervention can be considered the definitive diagnostic studies. Nevertheless, current practice has evolved away from the use of these methods to screen for and predict benefit in patients with renovascular disease. The following discussion will center on currently used screening tests and indications for intervention in the treatment of renovascular disease.

CURRENT CONCEPTS IN DIAGNOSTIC STUDIES

Identification of a noninvasive screening test that will identify accurately all patients with renovascular disease who might require interventional management remains an elusive goal. Prior methods such as peripheral plasma renin activity, rapid-sequence intravenous pyelography, and saralasin infusion are examples of such tests that have been abandoned. Isotope renography continues to be proposed as a valuable screening test, yet the methods employed are being modified continuously with the hope of improving the sensitivity and specificity. The newest versions of isotope renography consist of renal scans performed before and after exercise or captopril infusion.[15] In these methods, a test is interpreted as positive when there is augmentation of derangements in renal perfusion following exercise or captopril infusion. Although these methods have improved the specificity of isotope renography, their reliance on activation of the renin-angiotensin system leads to an unacceptable incidence of false-negative results.

Furthermore, interpretation of the renogram after captopril infusion requires its comparison to a relatively normal baseline scan. Although this frequently is the case when the occasional young patient with fibromuscular dysplasia is being evaluated, a near-normal renogram is uncommon in our patient population, which is composed mostly of patients with ischemic nephropathy.

Our bias is that screening tests that image the vascular anatomy and assess the hemodynamics of renal flow are the most promising methods for widespread screening for renovascular disease. In this regard, vascular images using magnetic resonance imaging or positron emission tomography may hold great promise. Current expense, lack of widespread availability, and limitations of patient selection criteria prevent their application as screening tools except in the most unusual circumstances.

Renal duplex sonography (RDS) has been proposed by several investigators as a useful screening test with which candidates for arteriography can be identified. We have reported our experience with RDS and evaluated its sensitivity and specificity for identification of renovascular occlusive disease.[16] The study population for RDS validity analysis consisted of 74 consecutive patients who had 77 comparative RDS and standard angiographic studies of the arterial anatomy to 148 kidneys. RDS results from 6 kidneys (4%) were considered inadequate for interpretation. This study population contained 26 patients (35%) with severe renal insufficiency (mean serum creatinine: 3.6 mg/dL) and 67 individuals (91%) with hypertension. Fourteen patients (19%) had 20 kidneys with multiple renal arteries. The presence of renovascular disease was identified correctly by RDS in 41 of 44 patients with angiographically proven lesions, and was not identified in any patient free of disease. When single renal arteries were present (122 kidneys), RDS proved to have 93% sensitivity, 98% specificity, 98% positive predictive value, 94% negative predictive value, and overall accuracy of 96%. These results were affected adversely when kidneys with multiple (polar) renal arteries were examined. Although the end-diastolic ratio was correlated inversely with serum creatinine ($r = .30773$, $P = .009$), low end-diastolic ratios in 35 patients submitted to renovascular reconstruction did not preclude beneficial blood pressure or renal function response. We concluded from this analysis that RDS can be a valuable screening test in the search for correctable renovascular disease causing global renal ischemia and secondary renal insufficiency (ischemic nephropathy). However, RDS does not exclude polar vessel renovascular disease causing hypertension alone, nor does it predict hypertension or renal function response after correction of renovascular disease.

With these results in mind, we now use RDS as the screening tool of choice. Nevertheless, since it does not identify accessory vessels or branch vessel disease accurately, we will proceed to arteriography when hypertension is severe or difficult to control, or when it is occurring in pediatric-age patients.

Although intra-arterial digital subtraction angiography is used in many centers to evaluate the renal arteries, we have continued to use standard "cut film" arteriography. Our predominant reliance on standard "cut film" arteriography in patients with renal insufficiency requires comment. In our experience, adequate assessment of the renal vasculature and juxtarenal aorta requires multiple injections when intra-arterial digital subtraction angiography is used. A single midstream flush aortogram requires no more contrast material than is required for multiple intra-arterial digital subtraction studies. In addition, standard arteriography provides information concerning cortical thickness and renal length, as well as improved clarity for interpretation of the renal artery anatomy. The fact that arteriography in patients with severe renal insufficiency, especially those with concomitant diabetes mellitus, can aggravate renal failure is recognized widely. Nevertheless, we believe that this risk is justified in such patients who have severe or accelerated hypertension and in those with positive RDS results. In these circumstances, the potential benefit derived from the identification and correction of a functionally significant renovascular occlusive lesion exceeds the risk of arteriography.

Functional assessment of lesions found on arteriography remains an important component of the diagnostic evaluation. Unfortunately, erroneous results of poorly performed studies have led many individuals to abandon the use of such studies and to rely solely on "clinical judgment" to predict benefit from renovascular surgery. Although the use of clinical judgment is appropriate in many patients, we continue to use renal vein renin assays in the evaluation of those with unilateral lesions. As a standard rule, we will not recommend revascularization of unilateral disease unless renin values lateralize to the involved side. When severe bilateral lesions are present, we make the clinical decision for intervention based on the severity of hypertension and the magnitude of associated renal insufficiency.

CURRENT INDICATIONS FOR INTERVENTION

Indications for correction of occlusive lesions of the renal arteries have continued to evolve, yet remain controversial. Whereas some individuals might offer renal revascularization only to a young patient with a non-atherosclerotic lesion causing renovascular hypertension, others have extended their indications to the prophylactic management of all anatomically severe lesions without regard to their functional significance. This discussion, therefore, will focus on the author's viewpoint regarding current indications for interventional management of renovascular disease.

Classically, operation for renovascular disease has centered on the treatment of secondary hypertension, that is, renovascular hypertension. This continues to be the predominant reason for intervention. Recently, however, the potential for simultaneous retrieval of excretory function in some patients with combined hypertension and renal insufficiency has been recognized. These observations have renewed awareness of this functional consequence of renal ischemia and have led to coinage of the term *ischemic nephropathy*. By definition, ischemic nephropathy reflects the presence of anatomically severe occlusive disease of the extraparenchymal renal artery in a patient with excretory renal insufficiency. Interestingly, this sequel of renovascular disease may affect a much larger population than the group of patients with renovascular hypertension. Recognition of ischemic nephropathy and the value of its management has altered the population presenting for renal revascularization.[17] Comparison of the group of patients currently submitted to operation by the author to that reported 20 years previously[18] is summarized in Table 1. This comparison underscores the changing and aging of the population that is undergoing operation.

Although this author believes that correction of the underlying cause of hypertension or renal excretory dysfunction by renal revascularization is valuable, I do not believe that available data argue for the preemptive, prophylactic correction of such lesions. Prophylactic correction of renovascular disease implies that operation is undertaken before there have been any pathologic sequelae related to the lesion. Therefore, by definition, the patient considered for prophylactic renovascular surgery has neither hypertension nor reduced renal function. Correction of the lesion in such a normotensive patient with no renal dysfunction implies proof that a significant percentage of such patients will survive to the point that the lesion has caused hypertension or renal dysfunction and that preemptive

TABLE 1.

Comparison of Earlier Surgical Experience With Current Series

Study Parameters*	1961–1972†	1987–1991‡
Number of patients	122	200
Mean age (yr)		
NAs-RVD	33	38
As-RVD	50	62
Duration of hypertension (yr)		
NAs-RVD	4.6	11.2
As-RVD	5.1	15.0
Renal artery disease (%)		
NAs-RVD	35	21
As-RVD	65	29
Renal artery repair (%)		
Unilateral	80	60
Bilateral	20	40
Combined§	13	32
Renal insufficiency (%)		
Not dependent on dialysis	8	65
Dependent on dialysis	0	6
Graft failure (%)	16	3
Hypertension response		
NAs-RVD		
Cured	72¶	43
Improved	24¶	49
As-RVD		
Cured	53¶	15
Improved	36¶	75

*NAs = nonatherosclerotic; RVD = renovascular disease; As = atherosclerotic.

†Data from Foster JH, Dean RH, Pinkerton JA, et al: *Ann Surg* 1973; 177:755.

‡Data from current series.

§Combined aortic repair for occlusive or aneurysmal disease.

¶Hypertension response excluding technical failures.

correction is necessary to prevent the occurrence of a clinically important event for which the patient cannot be treated. To test this hypothesis, we will review currently available data on the natural history of renovascular disease and the results of operative management.

The first points that one should address are the rate of progression of anatomically significant stenoses to total occlusion and the rate at which lesions not causing adverse sequelae progress to functional significance. Data regarding the frequency of angiographic progression in our series of patients[19] and those of other investigators[20, 21] are summarized in Table 2. Progression of ipsilateral lesions occurred in 44% of patients, and progression to total occlusion during noninterventional follow-up occurred

TABLE 2.

Angiographic Progression of Atherosclerotic Lesions of Renal Artery

Mean Follow-up (mo)	Number	Ipsilateral Lesions		Contralateral Lesions
		Percent Exhibiting Progression	Percent Progressing to Occlusion	Percent Exhibiting Progression
29–35*	85	44	16	—
28†	35	—	12	17

*Data from Dean RH, Kieffer RW, Smith BM, et al: *Arch Surg* 1981; 166:1408–1415; and from Wollenweber J, Sheps SG, Davis GD: *Am J Cardiol* 1968; 21:60–71.
†Data from Dean RH, Kieffer RW, Smith BM, et al: *Arch Surg* 1981; 166:1408–1415.

in 12%. However, among our reported patients,[19] only one (3%) had loss of a previously reconstructed renal artery.

One must assume that anatomic progression of a lesion is necessary for the subsequent functionally significant manifestation of a previously "innocent" lesion. Therefore, renovascular hypertension will develop in only about 44% of normotensive patients with an anatomically significant lesion. If one also assumes that the subsequent development of renovascular hypertension is treated by drug therapy alone so that progression of the causative lesion continues, then the next issue to address is the frequency of resulting deterioration in renal function. Table 3 summarizes the data from our patients on this question. During a 15- to 24-month follow-up period, significant loss of renal function, as defined by at least a 25% decrease in glomerular filtration rate, occurred in only 40% of the evaluated 30 patients randomized to the medical side of our prospective, randomized trial comparing surgical and medical management of renovascular hypertension. Nevertheless, 13% of those patients who subsequently were submitted to operation following severe deterioration in renal function continued to exhibit progressive deterioration. There-

TABLE 3.

Changes in Glomerular Filtration Rate or Creatinine Clearance During Medical Management of Renovascular Hypertension

Change	Number Affected (%)
Decreased by 25% to 49%	11 (37)
Decreased ≥50%	1 (3)
No change ±24%	14 (47)
Improved ≥25%	4 (13)
Total	30 (100)

fore, of the patients with renovascular hypertension who originally were randomized to a drug therapy group, only 36% had the potential for prevention of loss of renal function by means of an earlier operation. Finally, one must consider how many of these patients who lose function during noninterventional management may have that function restored by a subsequent operation. Novick and colleagues[23] have reported that 67% of properly selected patients will have restoration of renal function by renal revascularization.

The impact of these respective issues on the potential benefit provided by prophylactic renal revascularization can be appreciated by examining the outcome in 100 theoretical patients with anatomically significant renal artery lesions who do not submit to operation until after loss of renal function has occurred (Table 4). Renovascular hypertension will subsequently develop in 44 patients. Sixteen (36%) of these 44 patients will experience a preventable reduction in glomerular filtration rate during follow-up. Nevertheless, restoration of function by a delayed operation will be obtainable in 11 of these 16 patients (67%). In theory, therefore, only 5 of the 100 patients considered for prophylactic intervention would have benefited uniquely by such preemptive intervention.

Finally, one should understand that such an operation has associated morbidity and mortality, which must be considered in any discussion of the merits of interventional management. The operative mortality associated with the surgical treatment of renovascular hypertension is about 1% in centers with large operative experience.[14, 21, 23, 24] Furthermore, the early technical failure rate probably is at least 5%, and about 8% of initially successful reconstructions will fail during follow-up.[25–28] Therefore, if 100 patients are subjected to renovascular surgery, the ultimate outcome will be adverse in 14 of them.

TABLE 4.
Theoretic Comparison of Risk to Benefit (100 Patients) in Prophylactic Renal Revascularization

Benefit/Risk*	Number of Patients (%)
Benefit	
Progression to RVH	44/100 (44)
Patients with RVH who lose renal function	16/44 (36)
Renal function restored by later operation	11/16 (67)
Renal function not restored by later operation	5/16 (33)
Unique benefit	5
Risk	
Operative mortality	1 (1)
Early technical failure	5 (5)
Late failure of revascularization	8
Adverse outcome	14

*RVH = renovascular hypertension.

Theoretically, then, preemptive prophylactic renal artery surgery alone could prevent irreversible adverse outcomes in only 5 patients, but would produce adverse outcomes in 14 patients. Therefore, we find no justification for prophylactic renal artery surgery, either as an independent surgical procedure or as an additional procedure performed in conjunction with infrarenal aortic surgery.

Anatomic disease in juxtaposition to an aortic reconstruction has led to an empiric and liberal approach to simultaneous renal reconstruction in many centers, yet the exercise of clinical judgment in the application of a selective approach to such combined procedures is more appropriate. A prerequisite for considering simultaneous renal revascularization is the presence of hypertension. If the patient is normotensive, then operation should be limited to the aortic procedure. If unilateral renal artery stenosis is found in a hypertensive patient, then simultaneous renal revascularization should be undertaken only when functional significance is demonstrated by positive renal vein renin assays or split renal function studies. The only exception to this approach is when the hypertension is either severe or poorly controlled and medications cannot be altered to obtain renin measurements. In these circumstances, renal revascularization is undertaken, even though the blood pressure benefit is less predictable.

When a patient has bilateral renal artery stenoses and hypertension, the decision to correct the renovascular disease simultaneously with correction of the aortic disease is based on the severity of both the hypertension and the renovascular lesions. When the two renal artery lesions are not similarly severe, but instead, there is severe disease on one side and only mild or moderate disease on the contralateral side, then the patient is treated as if only a unilateral lesion exists. If both lesions are only moderately severe (65% to 80% stenosis), then renal revascularization is undertaken only if the hypertension is severe. In contrast, if the lesions both are severe (>80% stenosis) and the patient has drug-dependent hypertension, then bilateral simultaneous renal revascularization is undertaken without concern for the results of renal vein renin assays. In fact, functional studies are not undertaken, because a lack of lateralization does not exclude the presence of renovascular hypertension.

When contemplating simultaneous correction of incidentally identified bilateral renal artery stenoses with correction of aortic disease, one should compare the patient's status to that of this characteristic presentation. Clearly, the indications for renal revascularization increase as the patient's presentation more closely parallels this picture. In such situations, concomitant renal artery repair at the time of aortic surgery is indicated to preserve function, with an improvement of hypertension being a secondary goal. Such indications seem justified despite the acknowledged increased morbidity and mortality of a combined operation.

In contrast to prophylactic renal revascularization, empiric intervention is appropriate under select circumstances. Empiric intervention implies that hypertension, renal dysfunction, or both are present, although a causal relationship between the renal artery lesion and the clinical sequelae has not been established. The specific circumstances in which such empiric intervention might be contemplated are summarized in the following discussion.

Revascularization of unilateral renal artery occlusive disease may be appropriate as an independent procedure in the presence of negative functional studies (i.e., renal vein renin assays or split renal function studies) when (1) hypertension remains severe and uncontrollable with maximal drug therapy, (2) the patient is relatively young and without significant risk factors for operation, and (3) the probability of technical success is greater than 95%. In these circumstances, correction of the lesion may be justified in order to treat all possible causes of hypertension before assigning such a young patient to a group with a rapid rate of cardiovascular morbid events during long-term follow-up. However, because the probability of blood pressure benefit is low in such a patient, morbidity from the procedure also must be predictably low. Although we have undertaken unilateral renal revascularization in patients with renal insufficiency who have not had positive functional tests, such procedures have been performed as a part of our clinical research study on the role of intervention in the treatment of ischemic nephropathy. We do not recommend this as a clinically proved therapeutic intervention.

REFERENCES

1. Goldblatt H: Studies on experimental hypertension. *J Exp Med* 1934; 5:347.
2. Smith HW: Unilateral nephrectomy in hypertensive disease. *J Urol* 1956; 76:685.
3. Freeman N: Thromboendarterctomy for hypertension due to renal artery occlusion. *JAMA* 1973; 157:1077.
4. DeCamp PT, Birchall R: Recognition and treatment of renal arterial stenosis associated with hypertension. *Surgery* 1958; 43:134.
5. Morris GC Jr, Cooley DA, Crawford ES, et al: Renal revascularization for hypertension. Clinical and physiologic studies in 32 cases. *Surgery* 1960; 48:95.
6. Hurwitt ES, Seidenburg B, Hainovoco H, et al: Splenorenal arterial anastomosis. *Circulation* 1956; 14:537.
7. Luke JC, Levitan BA: Revascularization of the kidney in hypertension due to renal artery stenosis. *Arch Surg* 1959; 79:269.
8. Howard JE, Conner TB: Use of differential renal function studies in the diagnosis of renovascular hypertension. *Am J Surg* 1964; 107:58.
9. Stamey TA, Nudelman IJ, Good PH, et al: Functional characteristics of renovascular hypertension. *Medicine (Baltimore)* 1961; 40:347.
10. Page IH, Helmes OM: A crystalline pressor substance (angiotensin) resulting from the reaction between renin and renin activator. *J Exp Med* 1940; 71:29.
11. Braun-Menendez E, Fasciolo JC, Lelois LF, et al: La substancia hypertensora de la sangra del rinon, isquemiado. *Revista Sociedad Argentina Biologia* 1939; 15:420.
12. Lentz KE, Skeggs LT Jr, Woods KR, et al: The amino acid composition of hypertension II and its biochemical relationship to hypertension. *Int J Exp Med* 1956; 104:183.
13. Tobian L: Relationship of juxtaglomerular apparatus to renin and angiotensin. *Circulation* 1962; 25:189.
14. Dean RH: Operative management of renovascular hypertension, in Bergan JJ, Yao JST (eds): *Surgery of the Aorta and Its Body Branches*. New York, Grune & Stratton, 1979, p 377.
15. Meier GH, Sumpio B, Black HR, et al: Captopril renal scintigraphy—an advance in the detection and treatment of renovascular hypertension. *J Vasc Surg* 1990; 11:770–777.

16. Hansen KJ, Tribble RW, Reavis SW, et al: Renal duplex sonography: Evaluation of clinical utility. *J Vasc Surg* 1990; 12:227–236.

17. Dean RH, Tribble RW, Hansen KJ, et al: Evolution of renal insufficiency in ischemic nephropathy. *Ann Surg* 1991; 213:446–456.

18. Foster JH, Dean RH, Pinkerton JA, et al: Ten years experience with the surgical management of renovascular hypertension. *Ann Surg* 1973; 177:755.

19. Dean RH, Kieffer RW, Smith BM, et al: Renovascular hypertension: Anatomic and renal function changes during drug therapy. *Arch Surg* 1981; 166:1408–1415.

20. Wollenweber J, Sheps SG, Davis GD: Clinical course of atherosclerotic renovascular disease. *Am J Cardiol* 1968; 21:60–71.

21. Perry MO, Silane MF: Management of renovascular problems during aortic operations. *Arch Surg* 1984; 119:681–685.

22. Schreiber MJ, Pohl MA, Novick AC: The natural history of atherosclerotic and fibrous renal artery disease. *Urol Clin North Am* 1984; 11:383–392.

23. Novick AC, Pohl MA, Schreiber M, et al: Revascularization for preservation of renal function in patients with atherosclerotic renovascular disease. *J Urol* 1983; 129:907–912.

24. Hunt JC, Strong CG: Renovascular hypertension: Mechanisms, natural history and treatment. *Am J Cardiol* 1981; 32:562–574.

25. Dean RH: Surgical management of renovascular hypertension, in Bergan JJ (ed): *Clinical Surgery International. Arterial Surgery*, vol 8. Edinburgh, Churchill Livingstone, 1984, pp 80–93.

26. Novick AC, Khauli RB, Bidt DG: Diminished operative risk and improved results following revascularization for atherosclerotic renovascular disease. *Urol Clin North Am* 1984; 11:435–440.

27. Dean RJ, Wilson JP, Burko H, et al: Saphenous vein aortorenal bypass grafts: Serial arteriographic study. *Ann Surg* 1974; 180:469–478.

28. Stanley JC, Ernst CB, Fry WJ: Fate of 100 aortorenal vein grafts: Characteristics of late graft expansion, aneurysmal dilatation, and stenosis. *Surgery* 1973; 74:931–944.

Changing Concepts in Techniques of Renal Revascularization

RICHARD H. DEAN, M.D.

O ver the past 2 decades, the introduction of new antihypertensive agents and percutaneous transluminal angioplasty has changed the attitudes of many regarding the role of surgical intervention for renovascular disease (RVD).[1, 2] New treatment alternatives combined with the increasingly older patient population that is seeking treatment for RVD have led many physicians to limit the use of surgical intervention to patients who have severe hypertension despite maximal medical therapy, those who have anatomic failures or disease patterns that are not amenable to percutaneous transluminal angioplasty, or those who have RVD that is complicated by renal excretory insufficiency (i.e., ischemic nephropathy).[3] As a consequence of these changing attitudes and treatment strat-

TABLE 1.

Twenty-Year Comparison of Techniques Used for Renal Artery Surgery

Surgical Technique	1962–1971 Series (%)*	1986–1991 Series (%)†
Aortorenal bypass	93 (67)	148 (51)
Saphenous vein	63 (68)	104 (70)
Synthetic graft	27 (29)	35 (24)
Hypogastric artery	3 (3)	9 (6)
Ex vivo reconstruction	0	19 (7)
Reimplantation	0	36 (12)
Thromboendarterectomy	19 (14)	89 (31)
Combined procedure‡	16 (13)	64 (32)
Nephrectomy	26 (19)	18 (6)

*Series included 122 patients and 138 kidneys.
†Series included 200 patients and 291 kidneys.
‡Combined procedures are simultaneous renal and aortic procedures.

Advances in Vascular Surgery, vol. 1.
©1993, Mosby–Year Book, Inc.

egies, the demography of the contemporary patient population also has changed.[4, 5] Currently, our patient population is characterized by the predominance of atherosclerotic RVD complicated by site-specific atherosclerotic organ damage and renal insufficiency.[6] Consequently, contemporary surgical management has evolved considerably from methods predominantly used in prior eras.

The change in operative approach that has occurred over the past 2 decades is underscored by a comparison of techniques used in a series I reported in 1973[7] to those used in our current series of 200 consecutive patients treated between 1987 and 1992 (Table 1). Notable in this comparison are the findings that no ex vivo reconstructions were performed during the earlier era. Many of those patients account for the 19% nephrectomy rate noted during that time. Similarly, the frequency with which thromboendarterectomy and simultaneous correction of aortic disease (combined procedure) is performed has more than doubled. Much of this difference reflects the older, more diffusely atherosclerotic population now receiving operative management.

CONTEMPORARY TECHNICAL CONSIDERATIONS

A wide variety of techniques are available for use in renal revascularization. These include aortorenal bypass, thromboendarterectomy, renal reimplantation, and extra-anatomic renal artery bypass. Since complete descriptions of these techniques are available elsewhere,[8, 9] only those aspects that represent more contemporary issues of technique will be discussed.

ROUTE OF INCISION

MIDLINE INCISION

We use a midline xiphoid-to-pubis incision for all renovascular surgery that is performed to correct atherosclerotic disease and for any renovascular procedure that involves simultaneous correction of bilateral fibromuscular dysplasia. Extension of the incision alongside the xiphoid provides 2 to 3 cm of proximal exposure that are not available when the incision is stopped at the tip of the xiphoid. This small extension places the renal arteries in the upper portion of the wound at a more readily visible site.

FLANK INCISION

We limit use of the lateral subcostal or flank incision to patients in whom unilateral branch repairs of fibromuscular lesions are required and to those in whom a hepatorenal or splenorenal bypass is planned. Although this exposure places the kidney and the renal artery branches in the center of the wound and allows easy visualization of the entire extraparenchymal vasculature, an even greater advantage is that it limits the amount of bowel mobilization that is necessary and, thus, speeds postoperative recovery. This approach is equally useful for an ex vivo procedure. When the RVD is proximal, however, we prefer the midline approach. In this instance, we believe that the added mobilization of the bowel is justified in order to achieve the widest possible exposure of the juxtarenal aorta.

EXPOSURE CONSIDERATIONS

We usually approach either renal artery through the base of the mesentery when proximal lesions are to be corrected. When unilateral branch lesions are to be corrected, we prefer to reflect the right or left colon medially and approach the vessels from a lateral direction.

When bilateral renal artery lesions are to be corrected, and when correction of a right renal artery lesion or bilateral lesions is combined with aortic reconstruction, we modify these exposure techniques. First, we extend the base of the mesentery exposure to allow complete evisceration of the entire small bowel, right colon, and transverse colon; in this exposure, the posterior peritoneal incision begins with division of the liga-

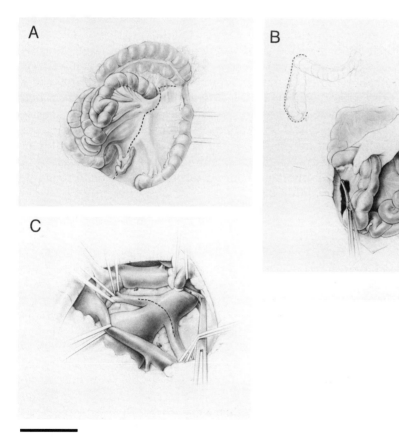

FIGURE 1.

Drawing of evisceration for bilateral renal artery exposure. The incision begins at the base of the mesentery **(A)** and continues around the cecum and up the right lateral mesocolon peritoneal reflection **(B)**. Through this technique, the entire small bowel and right colon is eviscerated for exposure of the juxtarenal aorta and both renal arteries **(C)**.

ment of Treitz and proceeds along the base of the mesentery to the cecum and then up the lateral gutter to the foramen of Winslow (Fig 1). Second, we extend the incision to the left along the inferior border of the pancreas to enter a retropancreatic plane, thereby exposing the aorta to a point above the superior mesenteric artery. Through this modified exposure, simultaneous bilateral renal endarterectomies, aortorenal grafting, or renal artery attachment to the aortic graft can be performed with wide visualization of the entire area.

One other technique we use occasionally is to divide partially both diaphragmatic crura as they pass behind the renal arteries to their paravertebral attachment. By this partial division of the crura, the aorta above the superior mesenteric artery is visualized easily and can be mobilized for supramesenteric cross-clamping.

AORTORENAL BYPASS

Three types of grafts usually are available for aortorenal bypass: autologous saphenous vein, autologous hypogastric artery, and synthetic prosthesis. Although the decision as to which graft should be used depends on a number of factors, we use the saphenous vein preferentially. If it is small (less than 4 mm in diameter), however, the hypogastric artery or a synthetic prosthesis may be preferable. We will use preferentially a 6-mm polytetrafluoroethylene graft when we are correcting proximal disease with a bypass and the distal renal artery is of large caliber.

We limit the use of hypogastric artery to aortorenal grafts in children. The saphenous vein has a tendency toward aneurysmal degeneration in this age group. For this reason, it should not be used for main renal artery reconstruction in children.

THROMBOENDARTERECTOMY

Thromboendarterectomy is used only for atherosclerotic renal artery stenosis. It is not applicable in fibromuscular disease. Transaortic endarterectomy of bilateral main renal artery lesions has been advocated strongly by Stoney et al.[10] In this procedure, the proximal aortic clamp usually must be placed above the superior mesenteric artery. If it is placed below this artery, it will seriously compromise the exposure of the orifices of the renal arteries. Visualization of the distal end of the renal artery endarterectomy, however, often is difficult or impossible with this procedure. Because of this, we prefer a transverse aortotomy, carrying the incision across the stenoses and into each renal artery. By this method, the entire endarterectomy can be performed under direct vision (Fig 2).

In either instance, however, we believe that postreconstruction intraoperative survey of the endarterectomized vessel with duplex sonography is extremely valuable. Through its use, residual lesions can be removed or distal intimal flaps "tacked down" via a separate renal arteriotomy.

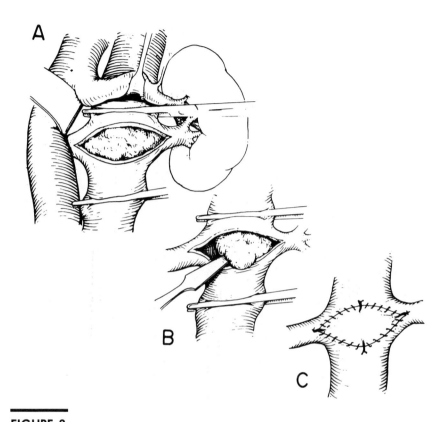

FIGURE 2.
A to **C,** drawing of arteriotomy for bilateral renal artery thromboendarterectomies.

EXTRA-ANATOMIC BYPASSES

An excellent description of extra-anatomic bypass procedures has been provided by Moncure and associates.[9] The use of hepatorenal, splenorenal, and iliorenal bypasses is gaining widespread popularity. I believe that these techniques should be reserved for a very small subgroup of high-risk patients and personally use them in less than 1% of my cases. In contrast to this viewpoint, extra-anatomic bypasses are being used increasingly as the primary procedure in lieu of direct aortorenal reconstructions. I believe that late follow-up of such liberal application of these techniques will confirm their inferiority as the standard procedure for renal revascularization.

EX VIVO RECONSTRUCTIONS

We employ ex vivo reconstructions when multiple branch lesions are to be corrected and special concerns regarding residual renal function are present (Fig 3). Several techniques are available for the performance of ex vivo reconstructions.[11, 12] Although some advocate routine autotransplantation,[13] we rarely find this to be necessary and most commonly place the kidney back into the renal fossa after ex vivo surgery. In performing

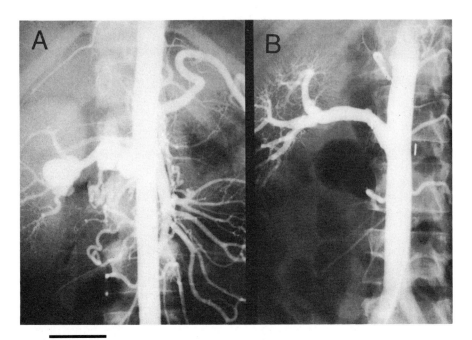

FIGURE 3.

A, preoperative arteriogram in a 25-year-old woman with a congenital solitary right kidney and multiple aneurysms of the right renal artery separately involving each of the branches. **B,** postoperative arteriogram after ex vivo repair and replacement of the kidney into the renal fossa.

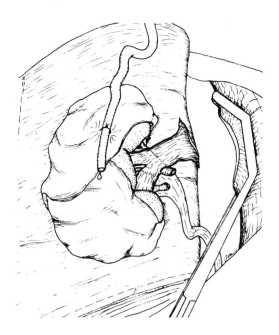

FIGURE 4.

Drawing of mobilized kidney and divided renal artery and vein for ex vivo repair. Note that a partial occlusion clamp is used on the lateral vena cava to excise an ellipse that includes the origin of the renal vein.

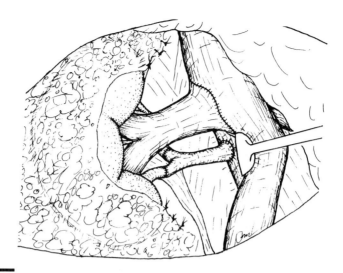

FIGURE 5.

Drawing of the reimplanted kidney with arterial and venous attachments completed. The envelope of Gerota's fascia is reattached to secure the kidney in its original position.

this technique, we remove an ellipse of vena cava that includes the renal vein organ (Figs 4 and 5). This technique protects against stenosis of the renal vein anastomosis. In addition, we do not perfuse the kidney continuously after removal. Instead, we believe that simple intermittent flushing with a chilled preservation solution provides equal protection during the shorter periods (2 to 3 hours) that are required for ex vivo dissection and complex renal artery reconstruction. For intermittent flushing, we refrigerate the preservative overnight, add the additional components (Table 2) immediately before use to make up 1L of solution, and hang the chilled (5 to 10° C) solution on an intravenous stand to provide a gravitational perfusion pressure of at least 2 m. Five hundred milliliters of solution is flushed through the kidney immediately after its re-

TABLE 2.

Electrolyte Solution* for Intermittent Flushing

Composition (g/L)		Ionic Concentration (mEq/L)		Additives at Time of Use to 931 mL of Solution
Component	Amount	Electrolyte	Concentration	
K_2HPO_4	7.4	Potassium	115	50% dextrose, 70
KH_2PO_4	2.04	Sodium	10	mL; sodium
KCl	1.12	Phosphate (HPO_4^-)	85	heparin, 2,000
$NaHCO_3$	0.84	Phosphate ($H_2PO_4^-$)	15	units
		Chloride	15	
		Bicarbonate	10	

*Electrolyte solution for kidney preservation supplied by Travenol Labs, Inc., Deerfield, Illinois.

moval from the renal fossa. As each anastomosis is completed, an additional 150 to 200 mL of solution is flushed through the kidney, a procedure that also reveals any leaks that may be present at the suture line.

Surface hypothermia is used to maintain constant hypothermia during ex vivo renal artery reconstruction. Our method of surface hypothermia consists of the following steps. We place 2-L bottles of normal saline solution in ice slush overnight. When we remove the kidney, we place it in a watertight plastic sheet from which excess saline solution can be suctioned away. We then place laparotomy pads over the kidney to keep it cool and moist by a constant drip of the chilled saline solution. Using this technique, we can maintain renal core temperatures of 10 to 15° C throughout the period of ischemia.

REFERENCES

1. Maxwell MH, Waks AU: Renovascular hypertension: Current approaches to management. *Pract Cardiol* 1987; 13:128–137.
2. Cumberland DC: Percutaneous transluminal angioplasty: A review. *Clin Radiol* 1983; 34:25–36.
3. Vaughan ED, Case DB, Pickering TG, et al: Indication for intervention in patients with renovascular hypertension. *Am J Kidney Dis* 1985; 5:A136–143.
4. Libertino JA, Flam TA, Zinman LN, et al: Changing concepts in surgical management of renovascular hypertension. *Arch Intern Med* 1988; 148:357–359.
5. Novick AC, Ziegelbaum M, Vidt DG, et al: Trends in surgical revascularization for renal artery disease. *JAMA* 1987; 257:498–501.
6. Hansen KJ, Ditesheim JA, Metropol SH, et al: Management of renovascular hypertension in the elderly population. *J Vasc Surg* 1989; 10:266–273.
7. Foster JH, Dean RH, Pinkerston JA, et al: Ten years experience with the surgical management of renovascular hypertension. *Ann Surg* 1973; 177:755–766.
8. Dean RH: Renovascular hypertension, in Moore WS (ed): *Vascular Surgery: A Comprehensive Review*, 2nd ed. Orlando, Grune & Stratton, 1986, pp 561–592.
9. Moncure AC, Brewster DC, Darling RC, et al: Use of the splenic and hepatic arteries for renal revascularization. *J Vasc Surg* 1986; 3:196–203.
10. Stoney RJ, Messina LM, Goldstone J, et al: Renal end-arthrectomy through the transected aorta: A new technique for combined aortorenal atherosclerosis. A preliminary report. *J Vasc Surg* 1989; 9:224–233.
11. Dean RH, Meacham PW, Weaver FA: Ex vivo renal artery reconstructions: Indications and techniques. *J Vasc Surg* 1986; 4:546–552.
12. Milsten R, Neifield J, Koontz WW: Extracorporeal renal surgery. *J Urol* 1974; 112:425–427.
13. Dubernard JM, Martin X, Gelet A, et al: Renal autotransplantation versus bypass techniques for renovascular hypertension. *Surgery* 1985; 97:529–534.

PART V

Status of Thrombolytic Therapy

Thrombolytic Therapy for Arterial Disease

MICHAEL BELKIN, M.D.

T he ability to lyse thrombus pharmacologically within the arterial system has offered an adjunctive treatment modality that has been accepted with enthusiasm by both vascular surgeons and interventional radiologists. As experience has grown, we have begun to understand the
benefits as well as the risks and limitations of this form of treatment. As
with many innovative forms of treatment, the initial wave of enthusiasm
and uncritical widespread application of thrombolytic therapy for arterial thrombosis has been followed by a leveling-off as indications have
become defined more clearly. The surgeon's perspective on the results of
thrombolytic therapy differs from that of the interventional radiologist because of our fundamental interest in long-term patency results as opposed
to the more short-term technical and radiologic results that are of more
immediate interest to the interventionalist. Nonetheless, most vascular
surgeons and interventionalists will agree that thrombolytic therapy has
assumed an established and important role in our armamentarium. In this
review, we will focus on the pharmacology of the fibrinolytic system and
the currently available thrombolytic drugs, as well as on ongoing research
on new agents as attempts are made to develop the "ideal agent." Advances in interventional techniques that have improved the safety, speed,
and completeness of arterial clot lysis in both the native vessels and bypass grafts, and the current accepted indications as well as contraindications for fibrinolytic therapy will be reviewed. The currently obtainable
short-term and long-term results will be discussed in some detail, as will
complication rates. Finally, an attempt will be made to distill this experience down to define the current recommended applications for thrombolytic therapy. Emphasis will be placed on the adjunctive rather than
competitive role thrombolytic therapy plays to surgical intervention.

THE FIBRINOLYTIC SYSTEM

There is a continuous and dynamic balance in the native circulation between factors causing thrombosis and those causing thrombolysis. The
simultaneous demands of fluidity within the circulation and hemostasis
at the site of injury require a precise mechanism to avoid either pathologic thrombosis or hemorrhage. Teleologically, therefore, it makes sense
that many of the factors that initiate the thrombotic cascade (such as activated Hageman factor) also activate the fibrinolytic system. The major

Advances in Vascular Surgery, vol. 1.
©1993, Mosby–Year Book, Inc.

components of the fibrinolytic system consist of fibrinogen, fibrin, plasminogen, plasmin, antiplasmins, plasminogen activators, and plasminogen activator inhibitors. A basic understanding of the role of each of these components is necessary to appreciate the mechanisms and side effects of exogenously introduced fibrinolytic agents.

FIBRINOGEN/FIBRIN

Fibrin is an autopolymerizing protein molecule that is formed as thrombin cleaves fibrinopeptides (A and B) from the circulating fibrinogen molecule. The fibrin is stabilized with covalent bonds and cross-bridges between molecules as the polymerization proceeds. Plasminogen as well as alpha-II antiplasmin is bound within the thrombus during fibrin polymerization. The binding of plasminogen within the forming thrombus plays an essential role in the fibrinolytic process.

PLASMINOGEN/PLASMIN

Plasminogen is formed by the liver as a 90,000-molecular-weight circulating globulin with 22 disulfide bridges. The plasminogen molecule contains five highly evolutionarily conserved looped structures called "kringles" that play an important role in binding to fibrin (Fig 1). Plasminogen exists in two basic forms. Glu-plasminogen (with a glutamic residue at its amino terminus) is incorporated more readily into polymerizing thrombus. Lys-plasminogen (with a lysine residue at its amino terminus) is formed as Glu-plasminogen is degraded partially by plasmin. Lys-plasminogen is activated more readily by exogenous plasminogen activators. The major step within the fibrinolytic system is conversion of the inactive plasminogen to plasmin, the active thrombolytic molecule. All plasminogen activators are serine proteases that cleave the arginine$_{560}$-

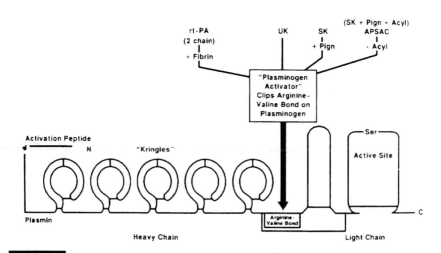

FIGURE 1.

Schematic representation of the plasminogen molecule and the site of plasminogen activation. SK = streptokinase; UK = urokinase; rt-PA = recombinant tissue plasminogen activator; $APSAC$ = anisoylated plasminogen-streptokinase activator complex.

valine$_{561}$ bond to create the two-chain plasmin molecule linked by disulfide bonds. The larger chain contains the fibrin-binding kringles, whereas the smaller chain contains the active proteolytic site. Plasmin is a nonspecific serine protease. Although fibrin is its main substrate, circulating plasmin will degrade other plasma proteins, including the various clotting factors. Physiologic fibrinolysis occurs as fibrin-bound plasminogen within the thrombus is converted to plasmin, thus activating the fibrinolytic system where it is most essential. Plasmin directly lyses the fibrin strands within the thrombus. As fibrinolysis proceeds, soluble fibrin degradation products are released and more plasminogen binding sites are exposed and filled, thereby perpetuating the formation of plasmin at the clot surface. The released fibrin degradation products may be measured in the plasma and have a variety of physiologic effects, including stimulation of hepatic fibrinogen release and anticoagulant properties that may persist beyond the period of active fibrinolysis.

As mentioned above, as thrombus is formed, plasminogen is incorporated within it. Thus, thrombus has incorporated within it "the seeds of its own destruction." As thrombus organizes and retracts, the intrathrombus plasminogen levels fall. This may explain partially the clinically recognized difficulty in lysing older thrombus.

PLASMIN INHIBITORS

As mentioned above, plasmin is a nonspecific serine protease with many plasma proteins, including clotting factors, as potential substrates. Thus, circulating plasmin free in the plasma may have several deleterious effects. Fortunately, a variety of effective circulating antiplasmins are available to bind and irreversibly inhibit circulating plasmin. The most important such inhibitor is alpha-II antiplasmin, which binds to plasmin in a 1-to-1 ratio. The second most important plasmin inhibitor is alpha-II macroglobulin, which binds to plasmin more slowly than does alpha-II antiplasmin and becomes important only when the latter is depleted. The efficiency of these antiplasmins is testified to by the extremely short half-life of free plasmin in the circulation (about 100 ms) and explains why exogenously supplied plasmin is an ineffective therapeutic lytic agent. Conversely, plasmin formed at the clot surface is relatively spared from antiplasmin inhibition and is able to lyse fibrin effectively. When exogenously supplied fibrinolytic agents (discussed below) are supplied, the antiplasmin system may be overwhelmed and the "systemic lytic state" may be observed. This manifests as a decrease in clotting factors, fibrinogen, plasminogen, and antiplasmin levels, as well as an increase in fibrin degradation products.

FIBRINOLYTIC AGENTS

All naturally occurring as well as synthetic plasminogen activators act by directly or indirectly converting plasminogen to plasmin via cleavage of the arginine$_{560}$-valine$_{561}$ bond. The ideal fibrinolytic agent would be one that forms plasmin only at the surface of thrombus, thus minimizing systemic effects. Unfortunately, even if such an agent were available, it would not be able to distinguish pathologic occlusive thrombus from physiologic hemostatic thrombus (such as that found at catheter entry or needle puncture sites). Other important qualities in an ideal agent include biocompatibility with minimal antigenicity or toxicity. The ideal agent would be easy to administer; have a short half-life, a reasonable expense, and a reliable dose response curve; and offer a predictable fibrinolytic response. There currently are four commercially available thrombolytic agents and several more are in development. Although each of these agents has particular advantages, none approaches the ideal qualities described above.

Streptokinase (SK) was discovered in 1933 when Tillett and Gardiner noted that the filtrate of group C β-hemolytic streptococci was able to lyse human clot in a test tube.[1] SK is a nonenzymatic, indirect activator that first must combine with plasminogen in a 1-to-1 fashion. This exposes an active site within the plasminogen molecule that in turn cleaves and activates other plasminogen molecules. SK was the initial agent used for intra-arterial therapy. Because it is a foreign protein, it is antigenic due to the ubiquitous nature of antistreptococcal antibodies in humans. This not only results in allergic reactions, but impairs the efficacy of the drug.[2] Neutralization of these antibodies with a loading dose of SK (250,000 or more units) has improved the lytic activity of this agent. Other disadvantages of SK include an unpredictable dose-response relationship and a significant activation of the systemic lytic state (even with local arterial infusions). Advantages of SK include its relatively low cost and the short half-life of the SK-plasminogen activator complex (18 minutes). Despite these advantages, the decreased efficacy and increased complication rates of SK have made other agents preferable for intra-arterial use.

Urokinase (UK) currently is the most commonly employed agent for intra-arterial use. Although urine long has been known to have fibrinolytic properties, it was not until 1946 that MacFarlane and Pilling isolated UK from urine.[3] More recently, the commercially available UK has been purified from human embryonic kidney cells maintained in culture. UK is a two-chain molecule that appears in two basic forms (molecular weight 54,000 or 33,000). Since UK is a human protein, it is nonantigenic. It is an enzymatic protein that directly converts plasminogen to plasmin. Because UK is a direct plasminogen activator, it has a more predictable dose-response relationship than does SK. It has a half-life of 16 minutes. The major disadvantages of UK include its relatively high expense and lack of fibrin specificity (i.e., it does not activate plasminogen selectively at the surface of thrombus). Despite these disadvantages, the improved safety and efficacy of UK over SK have made it the preferred agent for intra-arterial use.

Tissue plasminogen activator (tPA) is a relatively new agent with only limited reported use for intra-arterial therapy. As early as 1947, Astrup and Permin recognized the presence of a plasminogen activator in human tissue.[4] tPA originally was isolated from a human melanoma cell line and uterine tissue. More recently, recombinant DNA technology has allowed the isolation of an active form of tPA from an *Escherichia coli* carrier. The extensive research and development of tPA, as well as technical aspects of its production have contributed to its high cost. tPA is produced in a variety of active forms, single- or double-chain, with molecular weights ranging from 60,000 to 75,000. tPA has the shortest half-life (6 minutes) of currently available agents. A tremendous amount of interest has been paid to tPA because of its theoretical advantage of fibrin specificity. In the absence of thrombus, tPA is a relatively inactive plasminogen activator. The binding of tPA to fibrin, however, results in structural modification, greatly increasing the affinity of tPA for plasminogen. This theoretically increases the selective formation of plasmin at the thrombotic surface, thereby increasing clot lysis and decreasing systemic effects. Limited clinical experience with intra-arterial tPA has confirmed that it is a rapid and active lytic agent, but its theoretical fibrin specificity has not translated into decreased bleeding complications or decreased systemic effects of the infusion.

The newest commercially available fibrinolytic agent, anisoylated plasminogen-SK activator complex (APSAC), represents a novel modification of the SK molecule. The APSAC molecule is a complex of plasminogen and SK (i.e., the actual plasminogen-activating complex), with the active site blocked by in vitro acylation. When the complex is exposed to fibrin, deacylation occurs, thus forming active plasminogen activator. This strategy offers the theoretical benefit of fibrin specificity that SK lacks. This modification also has resulted in prolongation of the half-life of the agent from 18 minutes for SK to 90 minutes for APSAC. Although this prolonged half-life may offer an advantage for intravenous applications, a shorter half-life is preferable for intra-arterial use. Like SK, APSAC is antigenic due to the presence of antistreptococcal antibodies. As of this time, no significant experience with APSAC has been reported for intra-arterial use.

Intensive research is underway to develop new fibrinolytic agents that more closely approach the ideal. One such agent is scuPA or pro-UK. scuPA is believed to represent a single-chain precursor of the UK molecule. Although scuPA does not have as much fibrinolytic activity as UK, it does seem to demonstrate properties of fibrin specificity similar to tPA. Early clinical trials are underway and suggest potential benefits of this agent. Another strategy being explored is binding of fibrinolytic agents to fibrin-specific antibodies in an attempt to enhance fibrin specificity. Obviously, even the most fibrin-specific agents cannot distinguish pathologic from physiologic thrombus and, therefore, will be subject to hemorrhagic complications.

PLASMINOGEN ACTIVATOR INHIBITORS

The final major component of the fibrinolytic system is the plasminogen activator inhibitors. Two major inhibitors, PAI-1 and PAI-2, are produced by endothelial cells.[5] These proteins rapidly bind to and inhibit naturally occurring plasminogen activators. They play an important role in the ability of endothelial cells to modify and control the procoagulant and anticoagulant properties within the local circulation and, thus, maintain the essential balance between hemostasis and circulatory fluidity. It is unclear what role these plasminogen activators play when large doses of exogenous fibrinolytic agents are employed clinically. Nonetheless, ongoing research may allow us to modify the production of these inhibitors and further control the fibrinolytic process in pathologic states.

INTRA-ARTERIAL INFUSION TECHNIQUES

The original applications of fibrinolytic therapy for arterial thrombosis involved intravenous, systemic doses of SK. The low success rates and high complication rates rapidly led to the abandonment of this approach. In 1974, Dr. Charles Dotter, a pioneer interventionalist, was the first to employ intra-arterial SK through an angiography catheter.[6] His goal was to increase the speed and efficacy of clot lysis and simultaneously to decrease bleeding complications. He was only moderately successful (35% clot lysis, 24% bleeding). Interest waned until Katzen and Van Breda reported higher success rates with SK in 1981 (92% lysis, 17% major bleeding).[7] Results remained inconsistent until 1985, when Drs. McNamara and Fischer reported their series with a more aggressive infusion regimen employing UK rather than SK.[8] The infusion regimen they ultimately developed (or a modification of it) has become the standard protocol for most interventionalists.

In general, when fibrinolytic infusions are contemplated for either graft or native-vessel thrombosis, groin puncture should be performed in the contralateral extremity and a guidewire manipulated over the aortic bifurcation. This has the advantage of decreasing catheter-site hemorrhage. For more distal infusions, however, ipsilateral antegrade puncture may allow superior manipulation of the infusion catheter. When the site of thrombosis has been identified angiographically, the "guidewire traversal test" should be applied.[8] If a 0.035–outer diameter Teflon-coated guidewire may be passed easily through the occluding thrombus, rapid and complete thrombolysis may be anticipated. Conversely, failure of easy passage usually is predictive of a more protracted (and often unsuccessful) infusion. Some authors have combined a successful traversal test with an initial "lacing" of the thrombus with lytic agent.[9] This consists of an initial bolus of UK (100,000 to 250,000 IU) along the entire length of the thrombus. The goal of local infusion is to maximize the exposure of the surface of thrombus to the fibrinolytic agent. Most interventionalists have adopted a coaxial infusion system for this purpose. An inner catheter (usually 3-French) is passed through an outer sheath (usually 5- to 6.5-French). The inner catheter is imbedded within the thrombus, while the outer sheath is positioned at the proximal thrombus. The UK infusion then is split between the two catheters. In general, the infusion is initiated with 4,000 IU/min of UK and continued for 2 to 4 hours with a continuous infusion pump. At that point, angiography is repeated to assess the progress and the infusion is decreased to 1,000 IU/min. More or less aggressive infusion regimens may be adopted depending on the extent of lysis, the clinical response, and the presence or absence of complications. Angiography is repeated at 6- to 12-hour intervals until lysis is complete. With each subsequent arteriogram and documentation of further lysis, the inner infusion catheter and sheath may have to be advanced to maintain optimal exposure of the thrombus to the fibrinolytic agent. Patients receive concomitant full anticoagulation with heparin (partial thromboplastin time 2 to 3 times normal) via the proximal sheath. This has not increased bleeding complications appreciably, but has decreased significantly the incidence of pericatheter thrombosis. Patients are monitored in an intensive care unit (or other appropriate observation area) for vascular status, bleeding, and other complications during intra-arterial fibrinolytic infusion. Patient cooperation is an important part of a successful and safe fibrinolytic infusion. Patients are required to lie still on their backs or "log-roll" onto their sides. Patients who are unable to lie still and cooperate should not be considered candidates for intra-arterial fibrinolytic infusion. Serial hematocrit values as well as coagulation parameters are measured every 8 to 12 hours. Although prolongation of coagulation values does not correlate with efficacy, depletion of systemic fibrinogen below 100 mg/dL does correlate with the occurrence of bleeding complications. Naturally, the incidence of bleeding complications increases as the duration of fibrinolytic infusion increases. Therefore, we generally stop therapy when thrombolysis fails to progress over an 8-hour period between arteriograms. When thrombolysis is complete, we maintain anticoagulation with heparin until the lesion responsible for thrombosis is repaired.

More recently, several series have reported results using tPA as the fibrinolytic agent. Infusion techniques were similar to those used for UK. Graor and associates employed either 0.05 mg/kg/hour or 0.1 mg/kg/hour of tPA, whereas Meyerovitz and coworkers used a 10-mg bolus followed by 5 mg/hr.[10, 11] As will be reviewed below, this agent seemed to have a similar success rate to series using UK, although lysis seemed more rapid and bleeding complications were at least as high as with UK. A randomized trial currently is underway to compare the efficacy and safety of these two agents.

A variety of modified infusion regimens have been introduced recently in attempts to improve the speed, safety, and completeness of fibrinolytic therapy. The goal of all of these modifications has been to increase the exposure of thrombus to the exogenous fibrinolytic agent. One such modification is the use of multiple sidehole catheters for infusion of the fibrinolytic agent. This is especially helpful for long occlusions, in which multiple infusion sites maximize exposure of thrombus along the length of the occlusion. Another benefit of this technique is that less manipulation of the catheters is necessary to maintain contact with the thrombus. A second modification of the infusion technique involves the "pulsed-spray" method of infusion. With this technique, the lytic agent is infused through a special catheter as a pressurized jet into the surrounding thrombus. This results in clot maceration and theoretically increases the intrathrombus concentration of fibrinolytic agent. Preliminary results with this approach suggest that it significantly increases the rapidity of clot lysis.[12, 13] The final major area of interest involves modification of doses of fibrinolytic agent employed. Several investigators have theorized that higher doses of lytic agent will increase the efficacy of the lysing procedure and decrease the infusion intervals. It is hoped that shorter infusion intervals will increase the safety and decrease the cost of intra-arterial lytic infusions.

As mentioned earlier, the ideal fibrinolytic agent is not yet available and may never be achievable. Good patient selection and attention to technical aspects of intra-arterial fibrinolytic infusions, therefore, are the most important factors leading to successful and safe therapy. Although infusion protocols are important and serve as guidelines for therapy, it is impossible to overestimate the significance of the experience and expertise of the interventionalist. Seemingly small modifications in the infusion regimen or infusion catheter location may mean the difference between success and failure. As a corollary to this, the selection of fibrinolytic therapy for a particular patient may depend on the experience and skill of the particular interventionalist.

INDICATIONS AND CONTRAINDICATIONS

Intra-arterial fibrinolytic therapy has been employed successfully in a wide variety of thrombotic complications. The most widespread application is for acute native arterial thrombosis (either spontaneous or post—balloon angioplasty) or for thrombosis of arterial bypass grafts. Both prosthetic and vein bypass grafts may undergo successful thrombolysis. Although balloon catheter thrombectomy has been successful in restoring patency to thrombosed prosthetic bypass grafts, the long-term results of thrombectomy of vein grafts have been poor, with patency rates of only 19% to 28% 5 years after secondary intervention.[14, 15] This generally has been attributed to incomplete thrombus removal, as well as to trauma induced by the balloon catheter. The disappointingly low secondary patencies of thrombosed vein grafts after balloon catheter thrombectomy and revision have generated considerable enthusiasm for the use of fibrinolytic therapy. This interest has been fueled partially by a number of reports (reviewed below) that have documented an approximate 75% initial success rate in the thrombolysis of vein grafts. A number of theoret-

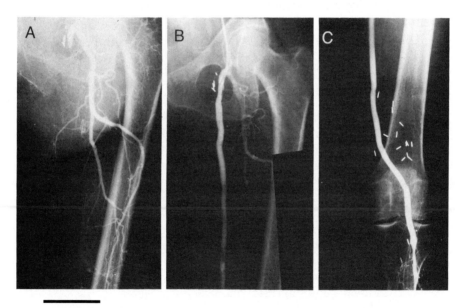

FIGURE 2.

A, the femoral arteriogram of a patient presenting with acute failure of a left femoropopliteal vein graft. **B,** visualization of the proximal portion of a patent popliteal vein graft after 16 hours of intra-arterial urokinase. **C,** arteriogram of the distal vein graft after thrombolysis showing severe progression of disease at the anastomosis and outflow track.

ical and practical advantages exist to the use of thrombolysis for this application. By lysing thrombus within the vein graft, intrinsic lesions of the graft may be identified angiographically prior to surgery, thus simplifying the graft revision. A second potential advantage of thrombolysis is more complete elimination of thrombus from both the vein graft and runoff bed than can be achieved with the balloon catheter. Finally, a third potential advantage is the avoidance of mechanical trauma to the vein graft that may be induced by the balloon catheter.

The intraoperative infusion of thrombolytic agents as an adjunct to balloon catheter embolectomy has received widespread attention recently. This generally has been done when outflow has been found to be compromised after restoration of perfusion. Techniques have not been standardized, and range from slow continuous infusions to large (250,000 units of UK) bolus infusions to extremely large doses using isolated limb-perfusion techniques. A number of small series have documented improvement in clinical status, arterial pulses, and arteriographic runoff. Because of the regional nature of the infusions and the limited half-life of the agents, surprisingly few bleeding complications have occurred as a result of this therapy. Although it is difficult to determine how much intraoperative thrombolytic therapy contributes in each case, it clearly has contributed to acute limb salvage in many patients.[16]

Whether fibrinolytic therapy is applied to either thrombosed native arteries or bypass grafts, successful lysis is able only to restore patency and define the lesion responsible for thrombosis. This underlying lesion then must be addressed surgically or with percutaneous transluminal techniques. Failure to correct the responsible lesion will lead predictably to rethrombosis. Figure 2 demonstrates the successful thrombolysis of an occluded femoropopliteal vein graft, revealing the progression of severe disease in the outflow tract and at the distal anastomosis. Long-term patency was achieved by an extension "jump-graft" to the peroneal artery.

The safe application of fibrinolytic therapy demands recognition of the contraindications to therapy. Most of these contraindications relate to the risk of hemorrhage during therapy. Table 1 lists the absolute and relative contraindications to systemic, intravenous fibrinolytic therapy. Although the risk of remote hemorrhage is higher with systemic therapy than with intra-arterial therapy, these contraindications should be considered when evaluating a patient for intra-arterial fibrinolytic infusion. Nonetheless, we have applied intra-arterial therapy successfully and safely in a number of patients with "relative" contraindications to systemic therapy. Because of the invasive nature of intra-arterial fibrinolytic therapy, several additional contraindications, not directly pertinent to systemic therapy, should be considered (Table 2). Because of the time interval necessary for intra-arterial fibrinolytic therapy to restore perfusion, the presence of severe ischemia with progressive neurologic changes should be considered an indication for surgery and an absolute contraindication to intra-arterial fibrinolytic therapy. Similarly, a devitalized limb with irreversible ischemic damage should not be subjected to fibrinolysis. Relative contraindications to intra-arterial therapy include the presence of a new Dacron graft (where transgraft hemorrhage may occur). Similarly, the infusion of grafts after early postoperative failure (<30 days)

TABLE 1.

Contraindications to Systemic Thrombolytic Therapy

   I. Absolute.
      A. Active bleeding source.
      B. Cerebrovascular accident within 2 months or other intracranial process.
  II. Relative (major).
      A. Recent major surgery or organ biopsy (within 2 weeks); postpartum status (within 10 days of delivery).
      B. Recent gastrointestinal bleeding.
      C. Recent trauma.
      D. Severe hypertension (>200 mm Hg systolic).
 III. Relative (minor).
      A. Recent minor trauma (including cardiopulmonary resuscitation).
      B. Left heart thrombus.
      C. Bacterial endocarditis.
      D. Coagulation deficits.
      E. Pregnancy.
      F. Hemorrhagic retinopathy.
      G. Active peptic ulcer disease.
      H. Recent streptokinase infusion (streptokinase only).
       I. Previous allergic reaction to streptokinase (streptokinase only).

TABLE 2.

Contraindications to Intra-Arterial Thrombolytic Therapy

   I. Absolute.
      A. Severe ischemia with neurologic changes.
      B. Devitalized limb with irreversible ischemic damage.
  II. Relative.
      A. Thrombosis of new Dacron graft.
      B. Acute postoperative graft failure (<30 days).
      C. Uncooperative patient.

may result in suture-line hemorrhage. In general, repeat exposure and thrombectomy is the safest and simplest approach in this setting. Finally, patients who are unable to lie flat and cooperate through the treatment regimen generally should not receive thrombolytic therapy.

RESULTS

Ultimately, the selection of intra-arterial therapy for any particular patient depends on a comparison of the risks vs. the benefits of this approach compared to alternative approaches. Such an evaluation demands knowledge of the results that may be anticipated with intra-arterial fibrinolytic infusion.

Critical assessment of the results of intra-arterial fibrinolytic therapy is complicated by the widely divergent definitions of a successful infusion, variation in infusion protocols, and different follow-up intervals. The criteria of a successful infusion may vary from complete clot lysis to recanalization with only "minimal" residual thrombus to simplify the establishment of antegrade flow through a thrombotic occlusion. Obviously, success rates will vary depending upon the stringency with which a successful infusion is defined. Similarly, the length of thrombolytic infusion necessary to complete lysis will vary with the timing of follow-up angiograms and catheter adjustments. More frequent interval angiography will establish the point of complete lysis in a more timely fashion than will less frequent angiographic monitoring. Furthermore, interventionalists and surgeons who demand complete clot lysis will require longer infusions than will those with less stringent expectations. Finally, the follow-up interval varies greatly among reported series. Most studies have defined success rates depending on the status of the patient at the time of leaving the angiography suite or being discharged from the hospital. More recently, several authors have begun to assess the long-term results of patients receiving intra-arterial fibrinolytic therapy. An appreciation of these long-term results is of fundamental interest to the vascular surgeon.

SHORT-TERM RESULTS

In general, short-term success rates of about 75% can be anticipated in reestablishing patency of thrombosed arteries or grafts (Table 3). In our experience, as well as that of others, UK has provided superior results over SK in achieving lysis.[17] UK has resulted in successful lysis in 60% to 100% of cases compared to 43% to 63% for SK. Despite its greater expense, increased efficacy and safety have made UK the preferred agent for intra-arterial therapy. More recently, several authors have reported their initial experiences with intra-arterial tPA. Gaor and colleagues reviewed their experience with intra-arterial tPA and reported successful lysis in 29 of 33 infusions (88%).[10] In another small (n = 32) randomized comparison of tPA and UK, Meyerovitz et al. noted similar success rates (50% for tPA, 38% for UK), but found faster lysis rates with tPA.[11] Bleeding complications with tPA appear to be similar or slightly higher than with UK. Thus, early results do not suggest any superiority of tPA over UK, although further studies are underway.

LONG-TERM RESULTS

When the long-term patencies of arteries and bypass grafts are reviewed after successful thrombolysis, the results are more sobering. We reviewed the long-term results of 22 occluded infrainguinal vein grafts that were lysed successfully and revised to correct the defects responsible for thrombosis.[20] Unfortunately, there was a high recurrent thrombosis rate, resulting in patency rates of only 37% and 23% at 1 and 3 years, respectively. Other authors assessing long-term patency results after lysis of vein grafts have noted similar results (Table 4). Parent and associates noted a 0% patency rate at 12 months after attempted lysis of nine autologous vein grafts.[21] Similarly, Eisenbud and coworkers found patency rates of only 17% 2 years after lysis of autologous grafts.[22] Two additional stud-

TABLE 3.
Short-term Results of Intra-Arterial Thrombolytic Therapy

Series	Drug*	Infusion Dose	Mean Duration (hr)	Number of Cases	Success Rate (%)	Number of Bleeding Episodes (%)
Belkin et al.[17]	UK	40,000 IU/hr	46	10	100	3 (25)
	SK	5,000 IU/hr	44	22	50	12 (55)
O'Donnell et al.[18]	UK	12,000 IU/hr	21	17	82	0 (0)
	SK	40,000 IU/hr	31	16	44	3 (19)
Gardiner et al.[19]	UK	60,000 IU/hr	26	22	77	1 (5)
	SK	5,000 IU/hr	47	22	41	5 (23)
Van Breda et al.[2]	UK	40,000–60,000 IU/hr	22	24	80	(8)
	SK	5,000–10,000 IU/hr	14	24	63	(33)
McNamara and Fischer[8]	UK	60,000 IU/hr	18	93	89	6 (7)
Graor et al.[10]	tPA	0.05–0.1 mg/kg	<8	22	88	9 (41)
Meyerovitz et al.[11]	tPA	10-mg bolus >5 mg/hr	—	16	50	5 (31)
	UK	60,000 IU/hr	—	16	38	2 (13)

*UK = urokinase; SK = streptokinase; tPA = tissue-type plasminogen activator.

TABLE 4.

Long-term Patency Rates After Successful Graft Thrombolysis and Revision

Author	Number of Grafts	Graft Type*	Follow-up Interval (yr)	Patency Rate (%)
Belkin et al.[20]	22	Vein	3	23
Parent et al.[21]	9	Vein	1	0
Eisenbud et al.[22]	15	Vein	2	17
O'Donnell et al.[18]	17	PTFE	2	37
Durham et al.[23]	41	Vein and PTFE	2	20
Graor et al.[10]	22	Vein and PTFE	1	20

*PTFE = polytetrafluoroethylene.

ies of combined infrainguinal vein and prosthetic grafts revealed equally disappointing results. Durham and colleagues noted only a 20% patency rate at 2 years (the median duration of patency was 162 days) after lysis of 41 vein and prosthetic grafts.[23] Likewise, in a series of 22 intrainguinal grafts (10 vein, 12 polytetrafluoroethylene), Graor and coworkers found only a 20% patency rate at 1 year after successful lysis and revision.[10]

The poor long-term patencies after thrombolysis of infrainguinal vein grafts may be explained by a variety of factors. One potential explanation may involve biologic changes that occur in the vein graft wall during thrombosis. Thrombin, for example, is a potent stimulator for the production of smooth muscle mitogens, which may contribute to progressive intimal hyperplasia.[24] The inflammatory or ischemic changes induced by thrombus may preclude long-term patency, despite the successful elimination of thrombus. Another potential explanation of the poor long-term patencies may be the advanced atherosclerotic disease of these patients and the poor general quality of their venous conduits. After successful lysis of vein grafts, we seldom identify a single area of stenosis in an otherwise high-quality conduit. Such grafts usually are identified by serial graft surveillance studies and are revised prior to thrombosis. Failed vein grafts generally are narrow conduits with extensive areas of stricture and hyperplasia. Attempts at revision of such grafts usually lead to suboptimal conduits with limited patency rates. In our experience, vein grafts that have failed in the early to intermediate postoperative period are more likely than late-failing grafts to have isolated defects that are favorable for repair.

One area in which the long-term results are more favorable involves the lysis of native arterial occlusions. Intermediate (15- to 24-month) patency rates have varied from 40% to 100%.[21, 22] Ultimately, long-term patency after thrombolysis of native vessels depends on the ability of the surgeon or interventionalist to correct the underlying lesion. The best results, therefore, may be anticipated when short segmental occlusions of large vessels are lysed. Figure 3 shows one such patient who progressed

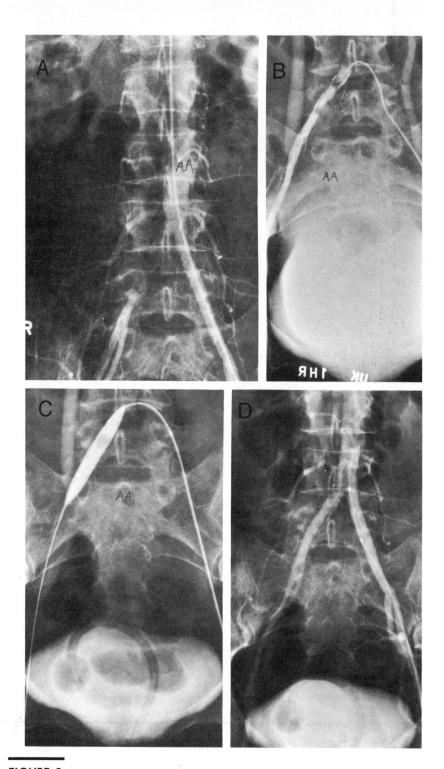

FIGURE 3.

A, aortoiliac arteriogram of a patient whose symptoms recently increased from claudication to rest pain. Arteriogram reveals segmental occlusion of the right common iliac artery. **B,** restoration of patency after 2 hours of intra-arterial uro-kinase. **C,** inflation of an intra-arterial balloon angioplasty catheter across the site of stenosis. **D,** the completion arteriogram revealing an excellent result of the PTA, which has been maintained for 2½ years.

suddenly from stable claudication to rest pain. Arteriography confirmed a common iliac occlusion, which was lysed successfully, revealing an underlying segmental stenosis. This underwent effective balloon angioplasty and remains patent 2.5 years later. We have had similar success in eight of nine patients subjected to thrombolysis followed by angioplasty of native vessels. As mentioned above, there are theoretical reasons why newer thrombotic occlusions will lyse more readily than older occlusions, and several authors have confirmed this clinically.[22, 23] Nonetheless, others have lysed successfully and angioplastied more chronic occlusions of the native vessels.[25]

ACUTE LIMB ISCHEMIA

Recently, several authors have become more aggressive in performing intra-arterial thrombolytic therapy in the setting of acute limb ischemia. There is some experimental evidence that thrombolytic infusion may increase the salvage of acutely ischemic skeletal muscle.[26] As mentioned above, however, due to time constraints, severe acute limb ischemia generally is considered a contraindication to thrombolytic therapy. Nonetheless, McNamara and coworkers have presented a well-documented series of 63 patients with acute ischemia (graded by Society for Vascular Surgery/International Society for Cardiovascular Surgery criteria) with 85% successful lysis and acceptable mortality (1.8%) and amputation (8.5%) rates.[27] It should be recognized, however, that these results were achieved by an experienced, highly skilled, and dedicated team of interventionalists. These results should not be generalized and, at this point, the application of thrombolytic therapy in this setting should be considered experimental.

COMPLICATIONS

The final factor in the selection of thrombolytic therapy is an understanding of the types and frequency of the various possible complications.

BLEEDING COMPLICATIONS

Given the therapeutic goal of thrombolytic therapy, that is, the dissolution of intravascular thrombus, it is to be expected that the most common, most feared, and potentially most serious complication of thrombolytic therapy is hemorrhage. Intra-arterial administration of thrombolytic therapy, by definition, requires continuous cannulation of the arterial system with an infusion catheter. Bleeding around the indwelling catheter or from the back wall of an arterial puncture site is by far the most common etiology of bleeding with intra-arterial therapy. Unfortunately, bleeding may occur anywhere that vascular integrity is compromised, resulting in central nervous system, retroperitoneal, urinary tract, vaginal, or aneurysmal hemorrhage, as well as in bleeding from almost any imaginable source.[28] As described earlier, plasmin is a nonspecific enzyme that may break down fibrinogen and other clotting factors. Depletion of these factors may result in an acquired coagulopathy. This coagulopathy may explain the observation that many bleeding complications occur after the cessation of thrombolytic therapy, when active clot lysis has stopped.

The incidence of significant bleeding is included in Table 3. Bleeding rates with SK have varied from 19% to 55%, whereas UK has been associated with lower rates of 0% to 25%. Early studies with tPA have reported bleeding incidences of 31% to 41%. Prolongation of the thrombolytic infusion and depletion of the fibrinogen level to less than 100 mg/dL are associated with an increased incidence of hemorrhage.

Minor bleeding at the catheter site is managed by simple compression. Major bleeding requires immediate cessation of the thrombolytic infusion. Resuscitation with crystalloid and packed red blood cells should be supplemented with fresh-frozen plasma (for clotting factors) and cryoprecipitate (to restore fibrinogen levels). In the setting of life-threatening hemorrhage, the plasmin inhibitor ε-aminocaproic acid (Amicar) may be infused to arrest fibrinolysis. The half-life of currently employed thrombolytic agents is short, however, and supportive measures almost always are adequate to maintain the patient through the active lytic phase. In our experience, the infusion of Amicar never has been necessary.

INTRA-ARTERIAL COMPLICATIONS

There are a number of complications of thrombolytic therapy that occur due to its invasive nature. Obviously, all the dangers inherent to angiog-

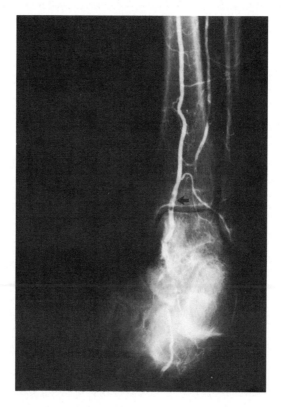

FIGURE 4.

A follow-up arteriogram taken during the course of intra-arterial thrombolytic therapy when the patient's ischemic rest pain increased. The arteriogram reveals the presence of intra-arterial emboli *(black arrow)* in the distal runoff bed. Continued lysis resulted in the resolution of these emboli.

raphy and arterial contrast also pertain to thrombolytic therapy. Pericatheter thrombosis was a major problem, but has been minimized by concurrent heparinization.[8, 17] When it does occur, it is managed by pulling back the infusion sheath and continuing the infusion.

As intra-arterial thrombus is lysed and blood flow is restored through the vessel, embolization of clot into the distal vasculature may occur. We have characterized the resulting clinical picture as "the storm before the calm," since these patients usually suffer an acute worsening of their ischemic symptoms that almost always resolves with continued infusion. Thus, when the patient suffers a sudden clinical deterioration and distal embolization has occurred, the reflex to discontinue therapy should be resisted. Arteriography may be useful in documenting the presence and extent of distal embolization (Fig 4).

SUMMARY AND RECOMMENDATIONS

The recommendation to employ thrombolytic therapy in a particular patient must be made on a case-by-case basis. On our service, there are very few "routine indications" for which we choose thrombolysis. The infusion of thrombolytic agents should be considered an adjunctive tool that the surgeon and interventionalist employ selectively to reach their goals in a particular patient. These goals may vary from achieving long-term relief from claudication in a relatively young, healthy patient to achieving a short-term solution in a patient with critical leg ischemia after a myocardial infarction. In some patients, the thrombolytic agent will be used primarily as a diagnostic tool. For example, a patient with a thrombosed vein graft and an acutely ischemic leg may have limited perfusion and no arteriographic visualization of the distal vessels. A short course of thrombolytic therapy may reveal a nonsalvageable vein graft, but also a patent distal tibial vessel suitable as outflow for a new bypass. In most cases, however, the thrombolytic infusion will be both diagnostic and therapeutic. For example, patency can be restored to a thrombosed artery or graft, allowing visualization and correction of the responsible deficit. Thus, given the myriad of clinical presentations and underlying pathologies, it is difficult to make firm recommendations that may be applied to all patients. The following simplified algorithms are designed as guidelines of the considerations we employ on our service.

SYMPTOMATIC ARTERIAL OCCLUSION

Our algorithm for applying thrombolytic therapy to symptomatic arterial occlusion is shown in Figure 5. Occlusions may be categorized as postprocedural or spontaneous. Immediate postprocedural occlusions, especially after transluminal balloon angioplasty, generally respond well to thrombolytic therapy. This is especially true when the occlusion is recognized while the patient is on the angiogram table. When a postprocedural occlusion is more delayed (for example, it occurs the day after a diagnostic arteriogram is performed), the best option may be thrombectomy or surgical reconstruction, as bleeding from the former puncture site may complicate thrombolysis. When symptomatic spontaneous atherosclerotic occlusions are identified with no recent major change in symp-

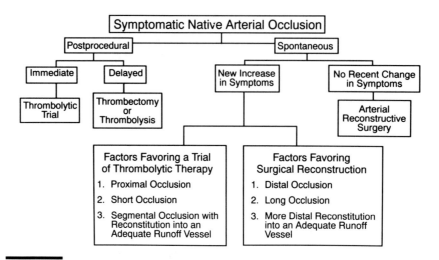

FIGURE 5.

Algorithm for applying thrombolytic therapy to symptomatic arterial occlusion.

toms, we proceed with surgical reconstruction if appropriate. If the patient has had recent onset or recent escalation of symptoms (suggesting recent thrombosis), we consider thrombolytic therapy. Factors that favor thrombolysis include a nonembolic, short segmental occlusion in a proximal vessel amenable to balloon angioplasty (such as the iliac artery). Other favorable factors include acute, extremely distal tibial or pedal occlusions and primary arterial thrombosis due to low-flow or hypercoagulable states. We tend directly toward surgical reconstruction for longer occlusions in the superficial femoral and popliteal arteries, which generally are managed better with bypass than with transluminal techniques. Similarly, we favor surgical thrombectomy for embolic occlusions, as thrombolysis of these organized emboli is not predictable and the surgical treatment is straightforward.

BYPASS GRAFT OCCLUSION

The algorithm for selection of thrombolytic therapy for thrombosed arterial bypass grafts is shown in Figure 6. If the patient has minimal or no symptoms, no intervention may be the most desirable option. The management algorithms diverge for prosthetic grafts and vein grafts. The short-term and long-term results for balloon catheter thrombectomy of prosthetic grafts have been acceptable. Furthermore, the lesions responsible for thrombosis generally can be identified and corrected at the time of surgery. We usually reserve thrombolysis for complicated cases of recurrent thrombosis when the etiology of thrombosis is unclear. Replacement of the graft (especially with a vein graft) may be the best option for recurrent thrombosis of an infrainguinal graft.

The application of thrombolysis to thrombosed vein grafts offers more potential benefit. Unfortunately, long-term results warrant caution against overzealous use. In general terms, it can be stated that the best long-term results will be achieved by replacing the thrombosed vein graft with a new venous conduit. This is especially true when the thrombosed vein graft was known to be of marginal size and quality.

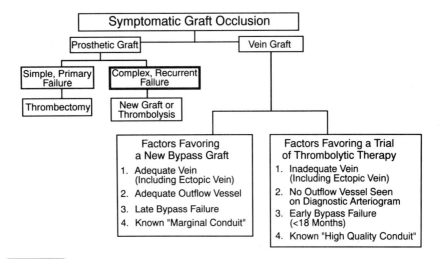

FIGURE 6.

Algorithm for selection of thrombolytic therapy for thrombosed arterial bypass grafts.

Several factors support a trial of thrombolytic therapy. Patients who present early (<2 days) after an early to intermediate occlusion (<18 months postoperative) of a vein graft are the best candidates for infusion, especially when their vein grafts were known to be of adequate caliber and good quality. Such grafts are more likely to have an isolated area of stenosis that lends itself to revision. We also select thrombolytic therapy for patients with insufficient autologous vein (including ectopic arm and lesser saphenous vein) for a new bypass graft. Thrombolysis may reveal a significant portion of the graft that can be salvaged, decreasing the need for additional vein. An aggressive posture must be taken to correct any and all graft defects if long-term success is to be anticipated. It should be recognized, however, that thrombolysis and revision of a failed vein graft may be only a short-term solution, with continued interventions being necessary to preserve limb salvage. An additional indication for thrombolysis of vein grafts is in patients in whom the arteriogram shows no outflow vessels suitable for bypass. A short course of thrombolytic therapy may reveal a patent distal outflow vessel, allowing construction of a new bypass.

REFERENCES

1. Tillett W, Gardiner R: The fibrinolytic activity of hemolytic streptococci. *J Exp Med* 1933; 58:485–502.
2. Van Breda A, Katzen BT, Deutsch AS: Urokinase versus streptokinase in local thrombolysis. *Radiology* 1987; 165:109–111.
3. MacFarlane R, Pilling J: Observations on fibrinolysis: Plasminogen, plasmin and antiplasmin content of human blood. *Lancet* 1946; 2:562–565.
4. Astrup T, Permin P: Fibrinolysis in the animal organism. *Nature* 1947; 159:681–682.
5. Schleef R, Loskutoff D: Fibrinolytic system of vascular endothelial cells: Role of plasminogen activator inhibitors. *Hemostasis* 1988; 18:328–341.

6. Dotter CT, Rusch J, Seaman AJ: Selective clot lysis with low dose streptokinase. *Radiology* 1974; 111:31–37.

7. Katzen BT, Van Breda A: Low-dose streptokinase in the treatment of arterial occlusions. *AJR Am J Roentgenol* 1981; 136:1171–1178.

8. McNamara TO, Fischer JR: Thrombolysis of peripheral arterial and graft occlusions: Improved results using high-dose urokinase. *AJR Am J Roentgenol* 1985; 144:769–775.

9. Sullivan KL, Gardiner GA, Shapiro MJ, et al: Acceleration of thrombolysis with a high-dose transthrombus bolus technique. *Radiology* 1989; 173:805–808.

10. Graor RA, Risius B, Young JR, et al: Thrombolysis of peripheral arterial bypass grafts: Surgical thrombectomy compared with thrombolysis. *J Vasc Surg* 1988; 7:347–355.

11. Meyerovitz MF, Goldhaber SZ, Reagan K, et al: Recombinant tissue-type plasminogen activator versus urokinase in peripheral arterial and graft occlusions: A randomized trial. *Radiology* 1990; 175:75–78.

12. Bookstein JJ, Fellmeth B, Roberts A, et al: Pulsed-spray pharmacomechanical thrombolysis: Preliminary clinical results. *AJR Am J Roentgenol* 1989; 152:1097–1100.

13. Kandarpa K, Drinker PA, Singer SJ, et al: Forceful pulsatile local infusion of enzyme accelerates thrombolysis: In vivo evaluation of a new delivery system. *Radiology* 1988; 168:739–744.

14. Whittemore AD, Clawes AW, Couch NP, et al: Secondary femoropopliteal reconstruction. *Ann Surg* 1981; 193:35–42.

15. Cohen JR, Mannick JA, Couch NP, et al: Recognition and management of impending vein-graft failure. *Arch Surg* 1986; 121:758–759.

16. Wyffels PL, DeBard JR, Marshall JS, et al: Increased limb salvage with intraoperative and postoperative ankle level urokinase infusion in acute lower extremity ischemia. *J Vasc Surg* 1992; 15:771–779.

17. Belkin M, Belkin B, Bucknam CA, et al: Intra-arterial fibrinolytic therapy: Efficacy of urokinase vs streptokinase. *Arch Surg* 1986; 121:769–773.

18. O'Donnell TF, Coleman JC, Santissi J, et al: Comparison of direct intra-arterial streptokinase to urokinase infusion in the management of failed infrainguinal ePTFE grafts, in Veith FJ (ed): *Current Problems in Vascular Surgery*, vol 1. St Louis, Quality Medical Publishing, 1989, pp 80–88.

19. Gardiner GA, Koltun W, Kandarpa K, et al: Thrombolysis of occluded femoropopliteal grafts. *AJR Am J Roentgenol* 1986; 147:621–626.

20. Belkin M, Donaldson MC, Whittemore AD, et al: Observations on the use of thrombolytic agents for thrombotic occlusion of infrainguinal vein grafts. *J Vasc Surg* 1990; 11:289–294.

21. Parent FN, Protrowski JJ, Bernhard VM, et al: Outcome of intraarterial urokinase for acute vascular occlusion. *J Cardiovasc Surg (Torino)* 1991; 32:680–690.

22. Eisenbud DE, Brener BJ, Shoenfeld R, et al: Treatment of acute vascular occlusions with intra-arterial urokinase. *Am J Surg* 1990; 160:160–165.

23. Durham JD, Geller SC, Abbott WM: Regional infusion of urokinase into occluded lower-extremity bypass grafts: Long-term clinical results. *Radiology* 1989; 172:83–87.

24. Daniel TO, Gibbs VC, Milfay DF, et al: Agents that increase cAMP accumulation block endothelial c-sis induction by thrombin and transforming growth factor-B. *J Biol Chem* 1987; 262:11893–11896.

25. Motarjene A: Thrombolytic therapy in arterial occlusion and graft thrombosis. *Semin Vasc Surg* 1989; 2:155–178.

26. Belkin M, Valeri R, Hobson RW: Intra-arterial urokinase increases skeletal muscle viability after acute ischemia. *J Vasc Surg* 1989; 9:161–168.

27. McNamara TO, Bonberge RA, Merchant RF: Intra-arterial urokinase as the initial therapy for acutely ischemic lower limbs. *Circulation* 1991; 83(suppl I):I106–I119.
28. Belkin M, O'Donnell TF: Complications of thrombolytic therapy, in Bernard VM, Towne JB (eds): *Complications in Vascular Surgery.* St Louis, Quality Medical Publishing, 1991, pp 433–441.

Appropriate Therapy for Acute Lower-Extremity Venous Thrombosis

ANTHONY J. COMEROTA, M.D.

SAMUEL C. ALDRIDGE, M.D.

Anticoagulation continues to be the standard therapy chosen by most physicians who treat acute deep venous thrombosis (DVT). Using pharmacologic or mechanical methods to treat DVT remains controversial. Reports demonstrate that lysis can be achieved with thrombolytic therapy, patency can be restored with operative techniques, and long-term postthrombotic sequelae can be reduced when either method is successful in clearing the deep venous system of thrombus. These observations have not been confirmed consistently, however, and many physicians are unwilling to risk the potential complications or encounter the additional expense associated with either thrombolytic therapy or venous thrombectomy. Although accumulated data demonstrate that significantly more patients regain patency of the venous system when they are treated with thrombolytic therapy compared to standard anticoagulation, in absolute terms, there are a substantial number of failures with lytic therapy. Therefore, individual physicians may not appreciate major advantages of thrombolytic therapy based on their own anecdotal experiences.

Preservation of venous function is the long-term goal of thrombolysis for acute DVT, and this includes regaining patency and maintaining valvular function. Those arguing against the use of lytic agents point to the risk involved, the cost of therapy, the limited application to only 15% to 20% of patients with DVT, and the low success rates reported in selected studies. Proponents of lytic therapy, however, emphasize that treatment today is less risky than quoted in earlier reports. They emphasize that the cost of the postthrombotic syndrome is exceptionally high, although it is spread over many years. Many patients with acute DVT are not candidates for lytic therapy, such as those in the early postoperative period or those with a history of intracranial disease. Many of the patients who are eligible are young and, therefore, likely to gain the greatest benefit from successful thrombolysis.

Available data documenting the results of thrombolysis potentially are biased, since, in many centers, lytic therapy for acute DVT is reserved for patients with the most severe disease (massive iliofemoral DVT/phlegmasia cerulea dolens). These patients are unlikely to respond to systemic

Advances in Vascular Surgery, vol. 1.
©1993, Mosby–Year Book, Inc.

thrombolysis because the iliofemoral venous system has extensive occlusion. Since venous flow is obliterated in the involved venous segments, it is unlikely that the plasminogen activator will reach the clot. In most medical centers, patients with less severe forms of acute venous occlusion, who are likely to have less severe postthrombotic sequelae, (but are more likely to respond to systemic lytic therapy), generally are treated with anticoagulants alone.

The underlying pathophysiology of the postthrombotic syndrome is ambulatory venous hypertension. The two important components producing ambulatory venous hypertension are residual venous obstruction and valvular incompetence. This was shown clearly by Shull et al.[1] when they reported their long-term observations after following patients who previously suffered acute DVT. In addition to the physical examination, they measured ambulatory venous pressures, performed ascending phlebography, and evaluated popliteal valve function. Their data indicate that valvular competence had the most significant impact on ambulatory venous pressures; however, venous obstruction was associated with higher ambulatory pressures for any given degree of valvular function. Therefore, the combination of obstruction and valvular incompetence was associated with the most severe ambulatory venous hypertension.

Killewich and colleagues[2] prospectively followed 21 patients with venous duplex imaging who had acute DVT treated with anticoagulation. Valvular incompetence developed in 13 of the patients (62%) during the 270 days following the acute episode. Interestingly, it took up to 3 months for some valves to become incompetent, and some patients developed incompetent valves in vein segments not involved with the thrombotic process. This new observation leads to the conclusion that the mechanism by which valvular incompetence occurs following DVT must involve more than just a physical effect of the thrombus on the valve.

Eight of the 21 patients (38%) did not develop valvular incompetence during the study. The majority who maintained good valve function long term had early and complete recanalization of the original thrombi (within 30 days). These observations suggest that early lysis of the thrombus preserves valvular function.

THROMBOLYTIC THERAPY FOR ACUTE DEEP VENOUS THROMBOSIS

The ideal management of patients with acute DVT should include (1) supportive care of the patient, (2) prevention of extension and embolization of the thrombus, (3) restoration of patency of the deep venous system, and (4) maintenance of venous valvular function.

Eliminating the thrombus can achieve the last three of these goals. Thrombolytic agents have been used in patients with acute DVT to this end. However, it is worthwhile to address several important questions in order to put the efficacy of thrombolytic therapy for acute DVT into proper perspective: (1) What is the natural history of anticoagulant therapy? (2) Can venous thrombi be lysed? (3) Is lysis of venous clot important for long-term valvular function?

Thirteen studies are reported in the literature comparing anticoagu-

TABLE 1.

Comparison of Heparin vs. Lytic Therapy for Deep Venous Thrombosis: 13 Studies*

Degree of Lysis	Percent of Patients	
	Lytic Therapy (n = 337)	Heparin (n = 254)
None/worse	37	82
Partial	18	14
Significant/complete	45	4

*Data from references 3 through 17. (Three papers are from a single institution and reported the same patients. References are inclusive; however, the patients are tabulated only once.)

lant therapy to thrombolytic therapy for acute DVT. Patients were evaluated with ascending phlebography initially and after therapy.[3-17] After pooling the data (Table 1), it was found that only 4% of patients treated with anticoagulants had significant or complete lysis, and that an additional 14% had partial lysis. The majority, 82%, had either no objective phlebographic clearing or actual extension of their thrombi. Therefore, only a minority of patients had sufficient clearing of thrombus to expect the return of normal venous valvular function. Among those patients treated with thrombolytic therapy, 45% had significant or complete clearing of the clot and 18% had partial clearing. Thirty-seven percent failed to improve or worsened.

Four additional studies describe the results of thrombolytic therapy for DVT, but were considered unsuitable for inclusion in the collective data base.[18-21] Two studies failed to include an anticoagulation cohort[18, 19]; therefore, comparative data were not available. Kakkar and Lawrence reported venous hemodynamic changes in patients followed for 24 months after initial randomization to treatment with streptokinase or heparin for acute DVT.[20] Unfortunately, the patients reported represent less than one third of those initially randomized and treated. It would be incorrect to assume that the response of those followed for 2 years is representative of all the patients initially randomized, since the initial results of therapy were not clarified in all patients, and since symptomatic patients are more likely to seek continued care than are those who feel well. It is possible that this report represents a pessimistic bias due to patient self-selection. Another study excluded from this tabulation was one performed by Schulman and associates,[21] who described the response of calf vein thrombosis to treatment with heparin or streptokinase. They reported treatment group response with an average quantitative venographic score, but failed to report individual patient response to therapy.

Two studies reported the long-term symptomatic results of anticoagulation compared to thrombolytic therapy following randomized treatment of the acute episode[13, 22] (Table 2). Although the follow-up period was shorter for the study by Elliot et al.[13] than for that by Arnesen et

TABLE 2.

Heparin vs. Lytic Therapy for Deep Venous Thrombosis: Long-Term Symptomatic Results*

| Agent Used | Number of Patients | Number of Patients with Postthrombotic Symptoms (%) | | |
		Severe	Moderate	None
Heparin	39	8(21)	23(59)	8(21)
Streptokinase	39	2(5)	12(31)	25(64)

*Data from Elliot MS, Immelman EJ, Jeffrey P, et al: *Br J Surg* 1979; 66:838–842; and from Arnesen H, Hoiseth A, Ly B: *Acta Med Scand* 1982; 211:65–68.

al.[22] (1.6 years compared to 6.5 years, respectively), both protocols were similar and used streptokinase. Posttreatment evaluation indicates that the majority of patients who were free of postthrombotic symptoms were treated with streptokinase, whereas most of those with severe symptoms of the postthrombotic syndrome received anticoagulation alone.

The most important question to be answered is whether lysis of deep venous thrombi preserves venous valvular function? In long-term follow-up of a prospective randomized study, Jeffrey et al.[15] have shown significant functional benefit 5 to 10 years after therapy of acute DVT in patients achieving successful lysis. The acute response to streptokinase therapy was similar to the pooled data reviewed previously. Patients then were followed long-term for popliteal valve incompetence and global venous insufficiency of the lower extremity using photoplethysmography and foot volumetry. Patients who had initially successful lysis were compared with patients who did not lyse, regardless of the therapy they received. Patients who lysed demonstrated normal venous function tests compared to significant venous insufficiency seen in patients who did not lyse. Nine percent of patients who had successful lysis had an incompetent popliteal valve, whereas 77% of those in whom lysis failed had popliteal valve incompetence. These differences were statistically significant (P<.001). Therefore, it appears that thrombolysis is preferable in those patients in whom it is not contraindicated.

Another important issue currently being evaluated is whether lytic therapy for acute DVT will reduce the incidence of recurrent DVT. The causes of failure of lytic therapy to regain patency of the deep venous system include poor patient selection, inadequate fibrinolytic response, and premature termination of therapy.

FAILURE OF THROMBOLYTIC THERAPY FOR ACUTE DEEP VENOUS THROMBOSIS

Patients with acute DVT who are selected for lytic therapy generally are those with the most extensive venous thrombosis, namely those with iliofemoral venous thrombosis or phlegmasia cerulea dolens. Since patients with extensive DVT are likely to have the poorest long-term outcome, this selection process represents an inherent bias when outcome evaluation is based upon the therapy given. In such patients, the venous system frequently is occluded by the thrombus, with no blood flowing through the involved veins. Therefore, plasminogen activators infused systemically will not reach the thrombus and cannot be expected to restore patency. Selecting patients with older thrombus also leads to failure, especially in patients receiving systemic infusion.

It has been demonstrated that the success of lysis is related to the amount of fibrin bound to plasminogen within the thrombus. The success of systemic therapy correlates with the age of the thrombus, and is poor in patients with a thrombus that is more than a week old. Unfortunately, clinicians cannot determine the age of a thrombus accurately and must rely upon the patient's symptoms for guidance. In many instances, however, symptoms and thrombus age may not be correlated closely.

All thrombolytic therapy is dependent upon the activation of plasminogen; therefore, systemic lytic therapy must be accompanied by a systemic fibrinolytic response. Failure to achieve adequate plasmin production is another reason for inadequate lysis.

Streptokinase has been the most frequently used plasminogen activator for the treatment of acute DVT. It is known that circulating antistreptococcal antibodies neutralize streptokinase, minimizing its fibrinolytic activity. Likewise, urokinase inhibitors also have been demonstrated. It is important that patients chosen for systemic lytic therapy be followed for appropriate fibrinolytic activation. Our practice is to obtain baseline coagulation studies, including a serum fibrinogen level. After beginning a systemic infusion, the partial thromboplastin time and fibrinogen level are redetermined at 6 and 12 hours, with a 25% or greater decrease in fibrinogen level anticipated with prolongation of the partial thromboplastin time. This indicates that a lytic effect is present and that the drug is activating plasminogen. The infusion is continued and the partial thromboplastin time and fibrinogen level are measured at 12-hour intervals. Although bleeding complications cannot be correlated precisely with laboratory studies of blood coagulation, we have found that patients demonstrating the most severe induced coagulopathy (i.e., fibrinogen less than 100 mg/dL) have the most frequent and severe bleeding complications. If profound hypofibrinogenemia occurs (<100 mg/dL), the lytic infusion is discontinued for 12 to 24 hours.

Discontinuing administration of the lytic agent before lysis is complete leaves patients with a residual thrombus burden and the continued risk of postthrombotic sequelae. In a prospective evaluation of 28 patients receiving thrombolytic therapy for acute DVT at Temple University Hospital, it was found that 36% had significant or complete clearing, 39% had partial clearing, and 25% failed to improve or actually worsened.[23] Patients were followed with sequential noninvasive studies every 12 to 24 hours for thrombus resolution. Venous duplex imaging is a reliable method with which to diagnose proximal DVT and follow its response to therapy. Ninety-five percent of patients who had a beneficial response demonstrated clot lysis within 24 hours of the initiation of therapy. Thirty-three percent of patients had their lytic therapy terminated while the clot was lysing. Of those patients with a partial response, 64% had the lytic agent discontinued while the clot was lysing but prior to maximal resolution. These data indicate that, in a substantial number of patients, therapy is discontinued prior to maximal lysis, and that this may be responsible for therapeutic "failure." Additionally, a predetermined duration of therapy may place the patient at higher risk of a bleeding complication if lysis occurs early and treatment is continued beyond the patient's maximal response. If the clot shows no lysis after 24 hours or completely resolves during this period, lytic therapy should be discontinued. On the other hand, if lysis occurs but is incomplete, lytic therapy should be continued until maximal lysis or resolution is documented.

CALF VEIN THROMBOSIS

Although most physicians agree that patients with proximal DVT should be treated, therapy for isolated calf DVT remains controversial. The controversy stems in part from studies involving noninvasive physiologic testing (i.e., impedance plethysmography, phleborheography). However, physiologic studies used for the diagnosis of DVT are inaccurate in asymptomatic patients. Additionally, physiologic noninvasive studies are unreliable for diagnosing calf vein thrombi and will not detect partially occluding thrombi, even if they are located in the proximal venous system.[24, 25]

The importance of definitive therapy for calf vein thrombosis has been clarified by the prospective, randomized study of Lagerstedt and colleagues.[26] They treated 51 patients with venographically confirmed calf vein DVT either with intravenous heparin for 5 days followed by a course of oral anticoagulation for 3 months or with the same heparin regimen followed by no anticoagulation. Patients in the heparin plus warfarin group had no recurrence during the 90 days of follow-up. In contrast, 8 patients (29%) in the group not receiving long-term anticoagulation had objectively documented recurrence. Of these 8 patients, 5 had proximal extension and 1 had a pulmonary embolus. Additional studies recently presented at an American Association of Orthopedic Surgeons meeting reported that asymptomatic pulmonary emboli were found in 6.8% of patients with calf thrombi compared to 1.7% of patients with negative phlebograms.[27] Symptomatic pulmonary emboli occurred in 1.7% of patients with calf thrombi and in only 0.2% of those with negative phlebograms.

In a study by Pellegrini and associates,[28] 11 patients with isolated calf vein thrombosis following total hip arthroplasty were followed, and none were treated following hospital discharge. Clots were located either in the muscular veins (6 patients) or in the axial deep calf veins (5 patients). No patient received anticoagulation following discharge from the hospital. Three of 5 patients with deep vein calf clots were readmitted for symptomatic pulmonary embolism, and 1 patient died. Based on these current data, and on data from the 1970s indicating that 20% to 30% of calf thrombi extend into the proximal veins, it appears that treatment of calf vein thrombosis is indicated unless the patient is at high risk for a bleeding complication. The latter patients should be placed in a careful surveillance program in order to detect proximal extension if it occurs. We have found frequent venous duplex examinations to be helpful, and will continue this surveillance until the high-risk period for thrombotic extension is over. The risk period does not necessarily end with hospital discharge.

There has been only one report of thrombolytic therapy for calf vein thrombosis.[21] Although lysis was demonstrated, it is difficult to determine whether these patients benefited compared with those treated with anticoagulation alone. The rationale for the use of lytic agents for calf DVT is that the majority of venous valves are located below the popliteal. We would consider lytic therapy for patients with calf DVT if it were extensive, involving the majority of the infrapopliteal veins. However, we have seen this only in patients who have undergone total knee replacement, who had contraindications to lytic therapy. A definitive study has not been performed and no data are available suggesting that any long-term benefit is achieved from thrombolytic therapy for acute calf vein thrombosis.

Based upon available data, we suggest that patients with calf DVT receive at least 3 months of anticoagulation, unless their risk for bleeding complications is high. If they are not treated, patients should be monitored with venous duplex imaging until the high-risk period has passed. If extension into the proximal venous system is demonstrated, the patient must be reevaluated for definitive treatment.

ILIOFEMORAL VENOUS THROMBOSIS

We have observed that patients with iliofemoral venous thrombosis who are treated with systemic lytic therapy frequently fail to recanalize and, therefore, have a disappointingly poor outcome. This also has been reported by others.[29] Failure to respond to systemic lytic therapy is understandable, since iliofemoral clot frequently is "packed" into the iliofemoral segment and has no exposure to flowing blood. Since the blood carries the plasminogen activator, very little of the activator reaches the thrombus. These patients require methods of delivery of the plasminogen activator different from those used in patients with the more routine forms of acute DVT. Venous thrombectomy plays an important role in the overall treatment scheme and should be used in conjunction with lytic therapy when indicated.

We believe that thrombolytic therapy can be successful if the drug reaches the clot. Therefore, direct intraclot infusion for patients with iliofemoral venous thrombosis and early phlegmasia cerulea dolens is our recommended approach. Ipsilateral intraarterial infusion with systemic doses of plasminogen activator has been given to patients with severe phlegmasia cerulea dolens and to those with early venous gangrene.

Prior to therapy, patients must be evaluated fully to clarify the extent of thrombus. The infrainguinal leg veins can be assessed accurately with venous duplex imaging. The proximal extent of the thrombus should be determined with phlebography, and the contralateral iliofemoral venous system and vena cava also should be studied phlebographically. This becomes important when alternative therapies are evaluated, since the contralateral iliofemoral segment may be used as the outflow system for the involved leg if residual iliac vein obstruction exists after lysis or thrombectomy. It also is important to document whether there is a clot in the inferior vena cava. If the patient has nonischemic iliofemoral thrombosis or early phlegmasia cerulea dolens, direct intraclot infusion is suggested. To accomplish this, a catheter sheath is placed in the contralateral femoral vein through which a guidewire and catheter can be threaded around the caval bifurcation into the common and external iliac vein thrombus. Alternative access through an ipsilateral femoral catheter or a transjugular approach can be used at the discretion of the physician. Use of the contralateral femoral vein allows placement of a vena caval filter, if indicated, prior to infusion. Although we have not used caval filters routinely for patients treated for iliofemoral DVT, we have inserted them in patients suffering acute pulmonary emboli with their current venous thrombotic episode and in patients with thrombus extending into the vena cava.

Once a guidewire is positioned appropriately in the thrombus, a multi–side hole catheter is used to infuse systemic doses of the lytic agent. We have chosen to use urokinase, delivered as a 250,000 to 500,000-unit bolus followed by a continuous infusion of 250,000 units/hr. Repeat phlebography through the infusion catheter is performed at 6- to 8-hour intervals. Therapy is continued until maximal lysis is achieved. The iliac vein thrombi tend to lyse sooner than the most distal thrombi, due to the direct activation of fibrin-bound plasminogen. Venous duplex imaging is used every 12 hours to follow lysis of the infrainguinal clot and as much of the iliac venous system as is accessible to the ultrasound probe.

If the infusion catheter cannot be positioned appropriately in the iliac vein thrombus, a venous thrombectomy is performed using current techniques,[28] which include complete operative and postoperative anticoagulation, on-table completion phlebography, and the creation of an arteriovenous fistula or cross-pubic venous bypass (if ipsilateral iliac vein obstruction persists). External pneumatic compression devices are used routinely postoperatively.

The details of our operative approach for iliofemoral thrombectomy are as follows. After establishing that the patient has iliofemoral venous thrombosis and after performing a contralateral iliocavagram to assess the status of the contralateral iliofemoral system and define the proximal extent of the thrombus, the patient is taken to the operating room. Regional or general anesthesia is preferred and standard blood salvage techniques are used, since blood loss easily can exceed 1,000 mL. A longitudinal incision is made over the femoral vein, exposing the common femoral, superficial femoral, and saphenous veins. A transverse venotomy is made cephalad to the saphenofemoral junction and the leg is elevated and compressed. Attempts at retrograde catheter passage are made to assist the thrombectomy of the leg, but usually are unsuccessful. A rubber bandage is applied from the foot to the thigh to assist with extrusion of the leg thrombus. A venous thrombectomy catheter is used to clear the iliofemoral venous system. Caval filtration or occlusion is not used routinely, since the likelihood of pulmonary embolism is small. If a caval filter is in place, the venous thrombectomy can be difficult, and must be performeᴅ with fluoroscopic guidance, using contrast material as the fluid with which to distend the balloon of the venous thrombectomy catheter. Intraoperative infusion of a lytic agent with balloon occlusion of the iliac

TABLE 3.

Scandinavian Randomized Trial of Thrombectomy Plus Arteriovenous Fistula vs. Heparin to Treat Iliofemoral Venous Thrombosis (6-mo Follow-up, n=63)*

Results of Treatment	Percent of Patients		
	Anticoagulation	Thrombectomy	P Value
Proximal patency	35	76	<.025
Patent femoral-popliteal segment with competent valves	26	52	<.05
Minimal/no symptoms	7	42	<.005

*Data from Plate G, Einarsson E, Ohlin P, et al: *J Vase Surg* 1984; 1:867–872.

vein can be used adjunctively. A small arteriovenous fistula is routinely created in an end-side fashion between the saphenous vein and the proximal superficial femoral artery. Since the saphenous vein usually is thrombosed, a proximal saphenous thrombectomy is required prior to creation of the arteriovenous fistula. Intermittent pneumatic compression is routinely used postoperatively to accelerate venous return from the leg. The poor results of venous thrombectomy reported 2 decades ago can be improved substantially with current techniques, as demonstrated by Plate and colleagues.[30] They performed a prospective, randomized study comparing venous thrombectomy with arteriovenous fistula to standard anticoagulation in patients with iliofemoral venous thrombosis. Operated patients showed significantly better patency and symptom-free outcome at 6 months compared to those treated with standard anticoagulation (Table 3).

Patients presenting with severe phlegmasia cerulea dolens or venous gangrene show signs of arterial hypoperfusion, and the question arises whether arterial or arteriolar thrombosis is occurring in addition to their severe venous hypertension. In such cases, ipsilateral intra-arterial infusion of thrombolytic agents has been used, placing the catheter into the ipsilateral femoral artery from the contralateral side. Infusing systemic doses of a lytic agent (urokinase, 4,000 units/kg/hr) with this technique ensures that the entire dose of the infused drug perfuses the involved leg. We have observed lysis of infrainguinal vein thrombi with a rapid drop in venous pressures associated with early symptomatic improvement following intra-arterial infusion. However, the thrombus in the iliofemoral segment persisted, most likely for the reasons mentioned previously. In this case, we have performed iliofemoral venous thrombectomy, although attempts at intraclot infusion are reasonable.

This combined approach to the patient with extensive iliofemoral DVT has been safe, showing no increased morbidity in patients so treated during the past 3 years. When venographically documented patency was restored, the early and longer-term results have been good.

SUMMARY

Patients who present with acute DVT should be evaluated and treated according to the location and severity of their disease. It is unfortunate, however, that, in some centers, all patients with acute DVT are treated in the same manner, whether they have minimal or extensive disease. Physicians have the optimal opportunity to clear the venous system pharmacologically early in the course of acute DVT, but the likelihood of successful lysis diminishes as time passes. The underlying pathophysiology of the postthrombotic syndrome and the natural sequelae of acute DVT make the goal of rapidly clearing the deep venous system of thrombus desirable. Pooled data from 13 phlebographically documented studies comparing recanalization of deep veins in patients treated with lytic agents to those treated with anticoagulation alone demonstrate significantly better clearance in those receiving lytic therapy. Few studies report follow-up data on their patients, and the results are inconsistent in those that do. However, patients treated with lytic agents appeared to benefit. If follow-up results are categorized according to the initial success of lytic therapy (i.e., actual clot lysis), patients treated successfully experience significant benefits compared to those not lysed successfully.

Modification of the method of delivering the plasminogen activator to patients with iliofemoral DVT to ensure high-dose infusion of the lytic agent to the thrombus should improve therapeutic outcome. We have used intra-arterial delivery of urokinase for massive phlegmasia cerulea dolens or early venous gangrene and direct catheter infusion into the iliofemoral clot in patients with less severe iliofemoral DVT. Both techniques can be used to significant patient advantage without compromising subsequent operative care.

Venous thrombectomy with arteriovenous fistula should be considered in all patients who are not candidates for lytic therapy, those in whom the catheters cannot be positioned properly, and those in whom lytic therapy fails. A large contemporary, prospective, randomized study demonstrates significant patient benefit compared to anticoagulation.

Patients with acute calf vein thrombosis should be evaluated and, if

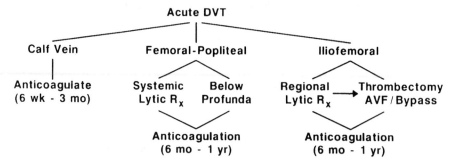

FIGURE 1.

Algorithm of preferred treatment (R_x) for acute deep venous thrombosis (DVT). This approach assumes that patients with calf vein thrombosis are not at high risk for anticoagulation and that patients with femoral-popliteal DVT do not have contraindications to thrombolytic therapy.

the risk factors associated with the onset of DVT have not been identified and eliminated, they should be treated or placed in a careful surveillance program. Current data indicate that anticoagulation is beneficial in patients with isolated calf DVT.

Patients with acute DVT should be stratified according to the severity and location of their disease. Advances in our understanding of anticoagulants, refined techniques of thrombolytic therapy, and the evolution of venous thrombectomy with its adjunctive measures all are available for use in appropriately defined patients (Fig 1). Matching the treatment to the extent of the patient's disease should substantially improve both the acute and long-term outcome of patients with acute DVT.

REFERENCES

1. Shull KC, Nicolaides AN, Fernandez JF, et al: Significance of popliteal reflux in relation to ambulatory venous pressure and ulceration. *Arch Surg* 1979; 114:1304–1309.
2. Killewich LA, Bedford GR, Beach KW, et al: Spontaneous lysis of deep vein thrombi: Rate and outcome. *J Vasc Surg* 1989; 9:89–97.
3. Browse NL, Thomas ML, Pim HP: Streptokinase and deep vein thrombosis. *BMJ* 1968; 3:717–721.
4. Robertson BR, Nilsson IM, Nylander G: Value of streptokinase and heparin in therapy of acute deep vein thrombosis. *Acta Chir Scand* 1968; 134:203–208.
5. Kakkar VV, Franc C, Howe CT, et al: Treatment of deep vein thrombosis: A trial of heparin, streptokinase and arvin. *BMJ* 1969; 1:806–810.
6. Tsapogas MJ, Peabody RA, Wu KT, et al: Controlled study of thrombolytic therapy in deep vein thrombosis. *Surgery* 1973; 74:973–977.
7. Duckert F, Muller G, Hyman D, et al: Treatment of deep vein thrombosis with streptokinase. *BMJ* 1975; 1:973–976.
8. Porter JM, Seaman AJ, Common HH, et al: Comparison of heparin and streptokinase in the treatment of venous thrombosis. *Am Surg* 1975;41:511–515.
9. Seaman JS, Common HH, Rosch J, et al: Deep vein thrombosis treated with streptokinase or heparin. *Angiology* 1976; 27:549–553.
10. Rosch JJ, Dotter CT, Seaman AJ, et al: Healing of deep vein thrombosis: Venographic findings in a randomized study comparing streptokinase and heparin. *AJR Am J Roentgenol* 1976;127:533–537.
11. Marder VJ, Soulen RL, Atichartakarn V: Quantitative venographic assessment of deep vein thrombosis in the evaluation of streptokinase and heparin therapy. *J Lab Clin Med* 1977; 89:1018–1022.
12. Arnesen H, Heilo A, Jakobsen E, et al: A prospective study of streptokinase and heparin in the treatment of deep vein thrombosis. *Acta Med Scand* 1978; 203:457–461.
13. Elliot MS, Immelman EJ, Jeffrey P, et al: A comparative randomized trial of heparin versus streptokinase in the treatment of acute proximal venous thrombosis: An interim report of a prospective trial. *Br J Surg* 1979; 66:838–842.
14. Watz R, Savidge GF: Rapid thrombolysis and preservation of venous valvular function in high deep vein thrombosis. *Acta Med Scand* 1979; 205:293–296.
15. Jeffrey P, Immelman E, Amoore J: Treatment of deep vein thrombosis with heparin or streptokinase: Long-term venous function assessment (abstract),

in *Proceedings of the Second International Vascular Symposium*. London, 1986, p 0.

16. Turpie AGG, Levine MN, Hirsh J, et al: Tissue plasminogen activator vs heparin in deep vein thrombosis. *Chest* 1990; 97:172S.

17. Goldhaber SZ, Meyerrovitz MF, Green D, et al: Randomized controlled trial of tissue plasminogen activator in proximal deep venous thrombosis. *Am J Med* 1990; 88:235–239.

18. Albrechtsson U, Anderson J, Einarsson E, et al: Streptokinase treatment of deep venous thrombosis and the post-thrombotic syndrome. *Arch Surg* 1981; 116:33–37.

19. van de Loo JCW, Kriessman A, Trubestein G, et al: Controlled multicenter pilot study of urokinase-heparin and streptokinase in deep vein thrombosis. *Thromb Haemost* 1983; 50:660–663.

20. Kakkar VV, Lawrence D: Hemodynamic and clinical assessment after therapy for acute deep vein thrombosis: A prospective study. *Am J Surg* 1985; 150(suppl):28–34.

21. Schulman S, Granqvist S, Juhlin-Danfelt A, et al: Long-term sequelae of calf vein thrombosis treated with heparin or low-dose streptokinase. *Acta Med Scand* 1986; 219:349–353.

22. Arnesen H, Hoiseth A, Ly B: Streptokinase or heparin in the treatment of deep vein thrombosis: Follow-up results of a prospective study. *Acta Med Scand* 1982; 211:65–68.

23. Comerota AJ, Katz ML, White JV: Thrombolytic therapy for acute DVT: How much is enough. *Circulation,* in press.

24. Comerota AJ, Katz ML, Grossi RJ, et al: The comparative value of noninvasive testing for diagnosis and surveillance of deep vein thrombosis. *J Vasc Surg* 1988; 7:40–49.

25. Comerota AJ, Katz ML, Greenwald LL, et al: Venous duplex imaging: Should it replace hemodynamic tests for DVT. *J Vasc Surg* 1990; 11:53–61.

26. Lagerstedt CI, Olsson CG, Fagher BO, et al: Need for long-term anticoagulant treatment in symptomatic calf vein thrombosis. *Lancet* 1985; 7:515–518.

27. Clifford B, Tribus CB, Haas SB, et al: Significance of calf vein thrombi after total knee arthroplasty. Presented at the American Association of Orthopedic Surgeons, San Francisco, March 1991.

28. Pellegrini VD, Francis CW, Harris C, et al: Embolic complications of calf thrombosis following total hip arthroplasty. Presented at the American Association of Orthopedic Surgeons, San Francisco, March 1991.

29. Hill SL, Martin D, Evans P: Massive vein thrombosis of the extremities. *Am J Surg* 1989; 158:131–135.

30. Plate G, Einarsson E, Ohlin P, et al: Thrombectomy with temporary arteriovenous fistula: The treatment of choice in iliofemoral venous thrombosis. *J Vasc Surg* 1984; 1:867–872.

PART VI

Issues in Basic Science

Hypercoagulable States in Patients With Peripheral Vascular Disease

MAGRUDER C. DONALDSON, M.D.

The ability of blood to coagulate is fundamental to bodily economy and homeostasis, and is a normal accompaniment of the response to stress, trauma, and inflammation. The delicate balance between coagulation in support of health and pathologic thrombosis contributing to illness involves complex interactions among circulating humoral and formed elements of the blood and the vessel walls. The conceptual framework for pathologic thrombosis established by Rudolph Virchow consisting of his famous triad of stasis of blood flow, vascular wall injury, and hypercoagulability remains helpful today. Although his studies and subsequent progress have focused largely on abnormal coagulation in the venous system, it has become clear that many of these same phenomena have an impact on the arterial side of the circulation. Thrombosis is the final common pathway for myocardial infarction, stroke, and peripheral arterial occlusion among patients with vascular disease in whom the "vessel injury" component of Virchow's triad is prominent, with unavoidable transient exacerbation by the modern techniques of surgery and interventional radiology. It is not at all surprising that a particularly high-risk subgroup of patients with vascular disease has emerged in whom the "hypercoagulability" component of the triad further enhances the risk of arterial thrombotic complications. The purpose of this chapter is to review advances in our knowledge regarding the hypercoagulable states and their impact on management of patients with peripheral vascular disease.

HYPERCOAGULABLE STATES

It may be convenient to conceptualize hypercoagulability as either (1) primary, with a specific, usually familial, abnormality; or (2) secondary, with a more complex, acquired abnormality (Tables 1 and 2).[1] Secondary hypercoagulability occurs as a physiologic accompaniment of stress and trauma, and also plays a prominent role in the pathophysiology of various disease processes. Most known hypercoagulable states first became evident in association with venous thrombosis. Definition of the role of hypercoagulability has been relatively elusive in patients with arterial disease, in whom multiple contributing causes of thrombosis usually coexist. In fact, both venous and arterial thrombotic complications related

Advances in Vascular Surgery, vol. 1.
©1993, Mosby–Year Book, Inc.

TABLE 1.
Primary Hypercoagulable States

I. Antithrombin III deficiency.
II. Protein C, protein S deficiency.
III. Fibrinolytic disorders.
    A. Hypoplasminogenemia.
    B. Abnormal plasminogen.
    C. Plasminogen activator deficiency.
IV. Dysfibrinogenemia.
V. Factor XII deficiency.
VI. Abnormal platelet reactivity.

to hypercoagulability usually occur only in the presence of one or more other predisposing risk factors. Thus, even though patients may have harbored a primary hypercoagulable state since birth, clinical manifestations may not arise for several decades when other circumstances such as pregnancy, surgery, or vascular disease become operative.

TABLE 2.
Secondary Hypercoagulable States

I. Abnormalities of coagulation and fibrinolysis.
    A. Malnutrition.
    B. Malignancy/chemotherapy.
    C. Nephrotic syndrome.
    D. Consumptive coagulopathy.
    E. Antiphospholipid syndrome.
    F. Pregnancy, use of oral contraceptives.
    G. Trauma/surgery.
II. Abnormalities of platelets.
    A. Myeloproliferative disorders.
    B. Paroxysmal nocturnal hemoglobinuria.
    C. Hyperlipidemia.
    D. Diabetes mellitus.
    E. Heparin-induced platelet activation.
III. Abnormalities of blood vessels and rheology.
    A. Stasis of blood flow.
    B. Hyperviscosity (polycythemia, leukemia, sickle cell disease, cryoglobulinemia/macroglobulinemia).
    C. Thrombotic thrombocytopenic purpura.
    D. Vasculitis, collagen-vascular diseases.
    E. Homocystinuria.
    F. Chronic peripheral vascular disease.
    G. Vascular trauma.
    H. Artificial surfaces.

CONGENITAL HYPERCOAGULABLE STATES

Most primary congenital hypercoagulable states result from abnormalities in the proteins that help regulate the thrombotic and fibrinolytic cascades (see Table 1). Quantitative deficiency of these proteins is most common, but mutant molecules that are dysfunctional also have been discovered. Both functional and quantitative antigenic assays are available for these proteins, but since defective mutant molecules may be detected by antigenic assay, resulting in normal total levels, the functional assay is a more physiologic measurement.

Antithrombin III (AT III) is a circulating anticoagulant synthesized in the liver that acts as a cofactor with heparin to bind and deactivate thrombin.[1, 2] AT III deficiency is inherited in an autosomal dominant heterozygous pattern and is the most prevalent of the congenital regulatory protein abnormalities, with an incidence of 1 per 2,000 to 5,000 in the general population. Homozygous inheritance apparently is incompatible with life. Patients with AT III levels below 60% of normal may exhibit resistance to heparin and are at increased risk of significant venous and arterial thromboembolism.[3]

Protein C is a vitamin K–dependent glycoprotein synthesized in the liver.[1, 2, 4] It is activated by thrombin, with greatly accelerated activation at the vascular intimal surface by the cofactor thrombomodulin. Protein C inhibits clot formation by inactivating activated factors V and VIII, and may enhance fibrinolysis by inhibiting tissue plasminogen activator inhibitor. Protein S is another vitamin K–dependent protein that functions as a cofactor for the anticoagulant activities of protein C.[5] Patients with autosomal dominant homozygous inheritance of protein C deficiency develop venous thrombotic complications very early in life. Heterozygotes without thrombosis and with 25% to 50% of normal protein C levels may occur in as many as 1 per 200 to 300 unselected blood donors,[6] with thromboembolism if additional risk factors develop. There are few reported cases of primary arterial thromboembolism related solely to familial protein C or protein S deficiency.[3]

Congenital dysfibrinogenemia has been recognized in which an abnormal fibrinogen molecule forms a fibrin gel that is resistant to normal removal by the fibrinolytic system. This abnormality may be detected by a prolonged thrombin time, and 10% of affected families suffer thrombotic complications.[7] Plasminogen deficiency or quantitatively normal but dysfunctional plasminogen detectable by immunoelectrophoresis occurs in association with both venous and arterial thromboembolism.[8, 9] There also is a rare familial defect in the release of plasminogen activator from vessel walls.[10] Finally, an apparent familial pattern of abnormal platelet reactivity has been described in association with arterial thrombosis.[11]

PHYSIOLOGIC ACQUIRED HYPERCOAGULABILITY

Pregnancy is associated with venous compression; increased plasma viscosity; increased levels of fibrinogen, factors VII, VIII, IX, X, and XII; and reduced levels of AT III and fibrinolytic activity.[1] As part of the normal homeostatic response to stress and injury, a stereotypic response follows major surgery, including vascular surgery,[12] with elevated levels of "acute-phase reactants," which include platelets and leukocytes as well as various plasma proteins such as fibrinogen, factor VIII, α_1-antitrypsin, plasminogen activator inhibitor, and antiplasmin. The transient reduction in fibrinolytic capabilities during the acute-phase reaction has been described as "fibrinolytic shutdown."[13] Platelets may become hyperreactive and AT III, protein C, and protein S deficiencies also frequently follow major surgery or trauma, further shifting the balance toward coagulation.[12]

PATHOLOGIC ACQUIRED HYPERCOAGULABILITY

Enhanced coagulability accompanies a host of pathologic conditions (see Table 2).[1, 2] Acquired AT III, protein C, and protein S deficiencies may occur because of decreased synthesis associated with severe liver disease and malnutrition, and because of increased loss with the nephrotic syndrome, massive thrombosis, and disseminated intravascular coagulation. Malignancy produces hypercoagulability in association with acute-phase reactants, tissue thromboplastin, fibrinolytic dysfunction, and lupus anticoagulant, as well as by activation of platelets by tumor cells and the production of procoagulant proteins by mononuclear and tumor cells. Chemotherapy can enhance coagulation by depression of regulatory protein levels as, for example, AT III deficiency caused by L-asparaginase. Hematologic malignancies and myeloproliferative disorders such as polycythemia vera increase viscosity and capillary sludging. Isolated thrombocytosis is not associated clearly with an increased risk of thromboembolism. Hyperlipidemia and diabetes have been associated with increased sensitivity of platelets to in vitro aggregation reagents. In addition, there is evidence of increased platelet thromboxane, decreased vessel wall prostacyclin, and increased platelet turnover in diabetics.[14]

Immune-mediated secondary acquired hypercoagulability has been recognized more frequently. Most prominent is the antiphospholipid syndrome (APS), in which a heterogeneous group of IgA, IgG, or IgM autoantibodies interferes with phospholipid-dependent biochemical reactions.[1, 2, 15–17] Among these reactions are the in vitro coagulation cascades measured by the partial thromboplastin time (PTT) and Russell's viper venom time (RVVT). Prolongation of these assays among a minority of patients with lupus erythematosus led to the term "lupus anticoagulant," broadened more recently to "lupus-like anticoagulant" upon discovery of the larger group of patients with normal PTT and RVVT but with specific anticardiolipin antibodies, present in 40% to 60% of patients with lupus. APS is associated with both arterial and venous thrombosis, and not with bleeding unless there is a coincident platelet or protein coagulopathy. The mechanism by which APS causes thrombosis is not clear, but increased platelet adhesiveness, decreased plasminogen activator release, and decreased endothelial prostacyclin production have been suggested. Though APS may occur with no overt signs of associated illness, it is present in many patients with lupus and other autoimmune or "collagen-vascular" disorders, cancer, and infectious diseases, and antibody levels may parallel waxing and waning of the underlying illness.

Heparin-induced platelet activation (HIPA) is an acquired hypercoagulable state present in about 6% of patients exposed to heparin.[18, 19] All types of heparin have been implicated. HIPA may be detected after intravenous or subcutaneous exposure and even after infusion of fluids through heparin-coated catheters.[20] Sensitized patients produce antibodies to platelet membrane antigens, resulting in enhanced platelet aggregation. Because rapid consumption of platelets results, a relative thrombocytopenia usually, but not always, occurs to a level below 100,000/mm^3. Thrombocytopenia may be noted as early as 4 days after the initiation of a daily heparin dosage, but may occur on the first day if the patient has had a previous heparin exposure. In addition to a falling platelet count, relative resistance to heparin may signal the presence of the antibody. HIPA may become undetectable in as few as 8 days, although it can persist for up to 28 months.[18] This phenomenon is distinct from the more common idiosyncratic thrombocytopenia that occurs in about 15% of patients within a few days of exposure and usually reverses during continuation of heparin.

HYPERCOAGULABILITY IN VASCULAR DISEASE

OVERVIEW OF THROMBOSIS IN VASCULAR DISEASE

In normal equilibrium, protein cascades, formed elements such as platelets and leukocytes, and the vascular wall interact in a complex balance governed by local and systemic hemodynamic and humoral phenomena. Prothrombotic factors maintain the integrity of the vascular compartment while opposing antithrombotic reactions and keep the blood liquid so it may circulate (Table 3).[21] For example, a break in the vascular lining resulting in exposure of the subendothelium initiates platelet adhesion, aggregation, and the release of granule products such as thromboxane, with concurrent generation of thrombin and production of a platelet-fibrin thrombus. Countering these normal prothrombotic events are antithrombotic reactants, including endothelial prostacyclin, AT III in conjunction with heparin-like substances in the vessel wall, protein C activated by thrombomodulin and working with protein S, and the fibrinolytic cascade initiated by endothelial secretion of tissue plasminogen activator. In addition, normal flow will act to minimize the size of the mixed plate-

TABLE 3.

The Intravascular Thrombotic Balance

Procoagulant	Anticoagulant
Damaged intima	Intact endothelium
Stasis	Normal flow
Tissue thromboplastin	Thrombomodulin/heparin cofactor II
Thromboxane	Prostacyclin
Prothrombin-thrombin	Antithrombin III, proteins C/S
Fibrinogen-fibrin	Plasmin-plasminogen
Plasminogen activator inhibitor	Plasminogen activator
α_1-Antitrypsin, antiplasmin	

let/fibrin clot at the vascular surface by diluting and sweeping away reagents and keeping most formed blood elements in the center of the laminar stream and away from the vascular wall. If shear is reduced by hypotension, local hemodynamic factors, or increased viscosity, reagents will congregate more readily at the site of injury and enlarge the thrombus.

The presence of disease in the vascular wall greatly compounds these phenomena by presenting irregularities that produce turbulence and hemodynamic alterations as well as unstable plaque, which may become disrupted, causing exposure of subintimal thrombogenic tissue, embolization, or abrupt vascular occlusion.[22] Indeed, there is evidence that chronic arterial disease is associated with ongoing thrombotic reactions most likely initiated at the vascular surface. For example, many patients with symptomatic cerebrovascular disease[23, 24] and myocardial infarction[25] have been found to have abnormally increased platelet reactivity. Patients with severe chronic peripheral vascular disease have elevated circulating levels of fibrinopeptide A, a by-product of fibrin generation, and β-thromboglobulin, a by-product of platelet granule release.[26] Markers of chronic thrombotic activity and platelet consumption are more pronounced in the presence of prosthetic graft surfaces.[27]

HYPERCOAGULABILITY IN PATIENTS WITH VASCULAR DISORDERS

Table 2 lists a substantial number of familiar conditions characteristic of many patients with vascular disease. Recent evidence has linked hypercoagulability to arterial thromboembolism in patients with vascular disease. For example, epidemiologic study has demonstrated a higher frequency of stroke[28] and myocardial infarction[29] in the morning hours of the day, with strong evidence associating this phenomenon with elevated circulating catecholamine levels and increased sensitivity of platelets to aggregating agents.[29] Though surgery and trauma long have been associated with venous thromboembolism, perioperative arterial complications such as stroke and myocardial infarction likely are related in part to such transient hypercoagulability.

Superimposition of unusual hypercoagulability is likely to have a deleterious impact on the success of revascularization. Endovascular injury, hemodynamic fluctuation, and systemic acute-phase responses are part and parcel of modern percutaneous and surgical therapy of vascular disease. In the immediate postoperative period, anatomic lesions such as intimal scrapes, plaque fractures, flaps, and retained valve leaflets present reactive foci on the luminal surfaces. Injudicious choice of inferior, small veins or extremely compromised outflow tracts introduces unfavorable hemodynamics. Mural hyperplasia associated with graft healing begins to have a gradual impact at sites of anastomosis, intimal injury, and residual anatomic defects. Finally, late disease progression eventually adds to the imbalance toward terminal thrombosis.[30]

The virulent nature of precocious vascular disease among young patients appears to be due in part to hypercoagulable states. In a study of 20 patients under the age of 51 years with severe leg ischemia, regulatory protein deficiencies or antiphospholipid syndrome were found in 45%, and platelet hyperaggregation was found in 47% of those tested.[31] Only 24% of the group had no detectable abnormalities. All 4 patients with early failure of infrainguinal grafts had proven hypercoagulable states. A similar study of 51 patients under the age of 40 years identified findings suggesting hypercoagulability in 6 of 8 patients with recurrent unexplained arterial thromboembolism, including thrombocytosis, AT III deficiency, and increased levels of factor VIII.[32] Three patients, aged 17, 19, and 42 years and members of a single family, have been described with abnormal in vitro platelet reactivity in association with arterial thrombosis.[11]

Defects in the fibrinolytic system have been found in patients with unexplained postoperative graft or spontaneous arterial thrombosis. A series of 8 patients, aged 21 to 57 years, was described in whom four venous and five arterial thromboses occurred.[33] Six of these patients suffered recurrent thrombotic episodes. All patients had normal antigenic levels of plasminogen and only 1 had an abnormally low functional level of plasminogen. Elevated levels of fibrinolytic inhibitors were detected in 4 patients. Immunoelectrophoresis against antiplasminogen sera revealed a band of material separate from normal plasminogen. The abnormal band was found in family members of 2 of the patients and in 10% of 30 control patients without evidence of pathologic clotting. A similar unusual immunoelectrophoretic band was found in 5 additional patients without atherosclerosis, aged 34 to 56 years, in whom extensive upper-extremity arterial thrombosis occurred spontaneously or after radial artery puncture, brachial artery catheterization, or arch aortography.[34] The functional plasminogen level was low in only 1 of these 5 patients.

AT III deficiency has been documented in association with unexplained spontaneous or postoperative arterial thrombosis.[35-37] In some instances, a history of previous thrombotic episodes suggested a congenital deficiency, and in others, the defect most likely was acquired. Serial AT III assays have shown a clear correlation between AT III, transferrin, and albumin, varying with state of nutrition and postoperative protein catabolism. Low AT III levels were found in 48% of patients with serum albumin levels less than 3.0 g/dL prior to vascular reconstruction. Early femorodistal bypass failure occurred in 33% of patients with low AT III levels and in only 13.4% of patients with normal levels.[38]

APS is associated with an increased incidence of spontaneous arterial thromboembolic complications in the cerebral and both upper- and lower-extremity arteries, occurring in patients who more frequently are young, female, and nonsmoking than in the general atherosclerotic population, with a high incidence of early thrombosis after bypass surgery.[16, 17, 39, 40] In a series of 18 vascular and 33 nonvascular surgical procedures in 23 patients with APS, 11 thromboembolic complications occurred in 4 patients, distributed among nine peripheral arteries, one coronary artery, and one venous site. Nine of the 18 vascular procedures were complicated by thrombosis and only 2 of the 33 nonvascular procedures were complicated. Steroids, aspirin, or anticoagulants appeared to confer protection against thrombosis after vascular procedures in this series.[41]

In a series of 455 in situ saphenous vein grafts, thrombosis within 30

TABLE 4.
Hypercoagulability Screening Panel

Laboratory Test	Normal Value
Regulatory proteins*	
Antithrombin III	75% to 120%
Protein C	60% to 125%
Protein S	60% to 140%
Plasminogen	80% to 120%
Antiphospholipid syndrome	
Russell's viper venon time	<30 sec
Anticardiolipin antibody	<22 IU
Heparin-induced platelet activation	Absent
Prothrombin time	
Activated partial thromboplastin time	
Thrombin time	
Hematocrit, white cell count	
Platelet count	
Erythrocyte sedimentation rate	

*Functional assays with results expressed as percentage of activity in control pooled plasma.

days of surgery occurred in 28 grafts (6.2%) due to 37 contributing causes, 8 of which (22%) were linked to evidence of hypercoagulability.[30] One failure occurred in a patient with proven HIPA, 1 in a patient with APS, and 1 in a patient with AT III deficiency. The additional 5 patients included 2 with associated systemic malignancy or collagen-vascular disease and 3 with clinical evidence of enhanced platelet reactivity producing the "white-platelet thrombus" phenomenon.

In a preoperative screening program designed to identify hypercoagulable states (Table 4), 272 vascular surgical patients underwent preoperative assay for AT III, proteins C and S, plasminogen, APS, and HIPA.[42] The results, which probably underestimate the actual incidence, since

TABLE 5.
Hypercoagulable States in 272 Patients with General Vascular Disorders

Hypercoagulable State	Number of Patients
Antithrombin III deficiency	3
Protein C deficiency	11
Protein S deficiency	4
Plasminogen abnormality	1
Antiphospholipid syndrome	18
Heparin-induced platelet activation	5

Total: 42 abnormalities in 37 patients (13.6%)

some patients were taking antiplatelet agents or sodium warfarin (Coumadin), demonstrated that 37 of the 272 patients (14%) harbored abnormalities (Table 5). Thrombotic complications occurred within 30 days of surgery in 11 (8%) of 137 of these patients, who subsequently underwent surgical revascularization, consisting of 5 infrainguinal graft thromboses, 2 myocardial infarctions, 3 cerebrovascular events, and 1 deep venous thrombosis. Within the group of 137 patients, 3 of 14 patients (21%) with documented hypercoagulable conditions sustained graft thrombosis, whereas only 2 failures (1.6%) occurred among the 123 patients with normal coagulation tests. Among the 3 infrainguinal graft occlusions associated with hypercoagulability, HIPA was present in 2 and APS was present in the other.

MANAGEMENT OF HYPERCOAGULABILITY

Successful management of hypercoagulability depends on accurate and timely diagnosis and therapy, at times under disadvantaged circumstances in which clinical judgment must be used without definitive laboratory support. Though they still are evolving, suggested algorithms for management are presented in Tables 6 through 8.

DIAGNOSIS

Given the potential deleterious impact of hypercoagulability on patients with vascular disease, it is worthwhile to attempt to identify prospectively such patients who may be at increased risk for intraoperative or early postoperative thrombotic complications. Evaluation should include a careful history and assessment of concurrent illness, focusing on past clotting disorders or the presence of one or more of the conditions listed in Tables 1 and 2. Patients younger than 45 years should receive particular attention, from the standpoint of both possible primary or secondary

---

TABLE 6.
Preoperative Management Strategy*

If:
   History of hypercoagulable state (see Table 1), predisposing illness or
      condition (see Table 2), or, previous unexplained thrombosis
   Age younger than 45 years
   High-risk reconstruction planned
   Elevated routine PTT, PT, HCT, WBC, platelets
Diagnosis:
   Hypercoagulability panel (see Table 4)
Therapy:
   (?) Alternatives to interventional therapy
   Preoperative aspirin
   Agents specific to condition (see Table 9)

*PTT = partial thromboplastin time; PT = prothrombin time; HCT = hematocrit; WBC = white blood cell.

TABLE 7.
Intraoperative Management Strategy*

If, < 1 hour after heparin:
  Routine ACT low
  Clot in wound
  "White thrombus" in reconstruction
Diagnosis:
  High ACT and normal/high platelet count—intimal injury
  High ACT and low† platelet count—HIPA
  Low ACT and normal/high platelet count—low AT III
  Low ACT and low platelet count—HIPA, low AT III
Therapy:
  Aspirin
  Intimal injury—revise segment; heparin/dextran, continue for 48
    hours
  HIPA—stop heparin; dextran, continue 48 hours; confirm diagnosis
    postoperatively
  AT III—supplemental heparin; fresh-frozen plasma

*ACT = activated clotting time; HIPA = heparin-induced platelet activation; AT III = antithrombin III.
†Platelet count >50,000 less than preoperative level.

TABLE 8.
Postoperative Management Strategy*

If no preoperative data and unexpected early thrombosis
Diagnosis:
  Exclude technical, hemodynamic cause
  Platelet count, HIPA assay
Therapeutic adjuncts to revision:
  Aspirin
  HIPA likely—alternatives to heparin (see Table 9)
  HIPA unlikely—heparin, dextran, consider postoperative sodium
    warfarin (Coumadin)
Confirm hypercoagulable state with postoperative panel (see Table 4)

*HIPA = heparin-induced platelet activation.

hypercoagulability and their precocious vascular diathesis. Routine laboratory evaluation should include prothrombin time, partial thromboplastin time, thrombin time, hematocrit, platelet count, and erythrocyte sedimentation rate determinations, with further assays as appropriate to confirm one of the known hypercoagulable states (see Table 4).

In addition to careful clinical evaluation and directed laboratory confirmation, we recommend preoperative screening of all patients with infrainguinal disease for APS and HIPA because of the apparent importance of these two acquired hypercoagulable states in this large subgroup. APS usually can be detected by a combination of Russell's viper venom time and anticardiolipin antibody. The most common assay for HIPA involves mixing the patient's platelet-poor plasma with pooled platelet-rich plasma in a standard aggregometer and observing aggregation upon the addition of heparin. Should HIPA be detected, the assay can be repeated, testing against patient or donor platelet-rich plasma after acetylation with aspirin to assess drug efficacy in vitro.[43] Since antiplatelet drugs may ablate HIPA, patients with negative HIPA results while on antiplatelet agents should continue to be treated until the risk of heparin exposure is over. In addition, HIPA should not be assayed while the patient is receiving heparin. Some investigators have suggested HIPA testing only if daily serial platelet counts fall while the patient is under heparin therapy,[19] relying on the fact that disastrous thrombosis is less likely to supervene if such vigilance leads to the prompt cessation of heparin.

Should unexplained thrombosis occur during or soon after vascular intervention, full investigation for the more frequent causes of hypercoagulability is warranted (see Table 4). Assessment of protein C and protein S levels is recommended, despite their apparent infrequent association with arterial thrombosis. Protein C, protein S, and AT III all may be reduced transiently during active thrombosis and in the perioperative period, so assessment should be repeated after recovery before concluding that a chronic deficiency exists. In addition, heparin reduces circulating levels of AT III,[44] and sodium warfarin (Coumadin) therapy will reduce proteins C and S since they are vitamin K–dependent. Tests for fibrinolytic inhibitors and platelet hyperreactivity, and immunoelectrophoresis to identify patients with abnormal plasminogen subspecies should be reserved for problematic patients in whom the other more common entities are found to be absent.

THERAPY

Optimal therapy of hypercoagulability includes general preventive measures designed to reduce the impact of stress, surgery, and intercurrent illness during the perioperative period. There is some evidence, for example, that epidural anesthesia and postoperative analgesia may reduce coagulability.[45] In addition, the importance of gentle, precise surgical technique aimed at protecting intimal surfaces cannot be overemphasized.

Routine preoperative therapy with antiplatelet or anticoagulant drugs is a reasonable strategy, with an acceptably low level of hemorrhagic morbidity as long as other unusual risk factors for bleeding are not present. Many experienced vascular surgeons rely on liberal use of these measures without attempting to screen patients vigorously preoperatively for hypercoagulable states, arguing that screening is imprecise, low-yield, costly, and usually results in the institution of the same preventive measures that would have been used in the first place. Our experience supports limited screening, since some patients suffer disastrous thrombotic complications despite broad antithrombotic measures, most particularly in the case of HIPA, in which heparin is contraindicated.

TABLE 9.
Therapy of Hypercoagulable States*

Fresh-frozen plasma
  Regulatory protein deficiencies (antithrombin III, proteins C and S)
Antiplatelet agents
  Aspirin for most patients with HIPA; APS for those with no clinically
    active other illness
  Iloprost as an intraoperative infusion with heparin in HIPA
Anticoagulants
  Heparin for all conditions except HIPA
  Dextran 40 as a perioperative substitute for heparin in HIPA and as
    an adjunct in high-risk circumstances
  Ancrod as a perioperative substitute for heparin in HIPA
  Warfarin (Coumadin) as a perioperative substitute for heparin in
    HIPA; as long-term therapy for APS with active associated disease;
    and as long-term therapy for chronic regulatory protein deficiencies
    and fibrinolytic abnormalities

---

*HIPA = heparin-induced platelet activation; APS = antiphospholipid syndrome.

We recommend routine preventive therapy with aspirin 300 mg daily starting prior to surgery or percutaneous intervention and continuing through the indefinite postoperative period. Patients at increased hazard for thrombosis because of the necessity for small-vessel reconstruction in the presence of other risk factors such as malignancy, malnutrition, hyperlipidemia, diabetes, or low-flow vascular prostheses probably should be treated also with intraoperative and postoperative low–molecular weight dextran (20 cc/hr) or heparin (500 to 750 units per hour) for a few days, though clear data on efficacy are not yet available.

Should specific hypercoagulable states be suspected or proven preoperatively, consideration should be given first to the use of noninterventional strategies to manage the patient's vascular problem. When postponement is not feasible or when unexpected thrombosis has led to the diagnosis postoperatively, specific therapy to correct the hypercoagulable state must be used (Table 9). Deficiencies in AT III and proteins C and S can be treated easily with replenishment using fresh-frozen plasma at the time of intervention and during early recovery.[37] Abnormalities in fibrinolysis are treated adequately by heparin followed by chronic sodium warfarin (Coumadin) anticoagulation.[33] Patients who have active collagen-vascular or other disease associated with APS may benefit from treatment of the primary illness using steroids, antimetabolites, or other appropriate medications in addition to anticoagulation with heparin followed by long-term sodium warfarin (Coumadin).[41] The presence of APS without an associated active clinical illness probably can be managed adequately with aspirin alone unless extra precautions seem warranted because of the presence of multiple other risk factors for thrombosis.

When HIPA is suspected, heparin should be avoided or stopped promptly while confirmatory testing is performed. If intervention can be postponed, most patients with HIPA will revert to normal within a few months provided they are not reexposed to heparin in any form during the interim.[18] The ill effects of HIPA may be blunted by perioperative aspirin in the majority of patients such that a single dose of heparin during vascular clamping often is possible under aspirin coverage despite the presence of HIPA.[46, 47] Alternatively, or if it is possible to demonstrate preoperatively that aspirin will not ablate in vitro platelet aggregation in the presence of heparin, a combination of sodium warfarin (Coumadin) started 1 to 3 days preoperatively and intraoperative low–molecular weight dextran (500 mL) is the most practical alternative to heparin when short clamp times are anticipated.[48] Among other options is the heparinoid, ORG 10172, which does not cause platelet aggregation in the presence of antibody.[49] The defibrinating agent ancrod also has been employed successfully as a surgical anticoagulant.[50] Another strategy consists of the use of the prostaglandin analog iloprost infused intravenously at the time of heparin administration.[43, 47, 48]

A number of studies have examined the impact of antiplatelet drugs on intermediate and late graft failure without regard to the presence of identifiable hypercoagulable states. No efficacy has been demonstrated for vein graft patency,[51] but there appears to be a small benefit for prosthetic grafts as long as the agents are started preoperatively.[52, 53] Most surgeons recommend indefinite postoperative aspirin administration because of the associated reduction in late myocardial events.[51, 54] Anticoagulation with sodium warfarin (Coumadin) also appears to have a beneficial effect on late patency of both vein grafts and prosthetics, though at the expense of a small but finite number of hemorrhagic complications. For example, a randomized, controlled trial demonstrated a significant improvement in 30-month cumulative graft patency among patients treated with sodium warfarin (Coumadin) after vein bypass for critical ischemia.[55] In another uncontrolled series of prosthetic grafts placed in infrageniculate positions, sodium warfarin (Coumadin) was associated with a 4-year cumulative primary patency of 37%, comparing favorably with reports of similar grafts without anticoagulation.[56]

CONCLUSIONS

It is clear that hypercoagulability has an important impact on the pathogenesis and management of vascular disease. Though vascular surgeons, relying on modern anesthesia, surgical technique, and antithrombotic agents, have been largely successful in controlling thrombosis, much remains to be learned about the complexities and varied conditions that lead to enhanced coagulability. Clinical data currently available must be expanded by sequential studies with control of physiologic variables as well as artifacts introduced by concurrent disease, surgery, medications, and laboratory methodology. Specific markers of the prothrombotic state and active thrombosis should be employed more widely in these investigations. It is highly likely that entirely new hypercoagulable states will be identified, offering insights into the unexpected thrombosis that regularly complicates the management of patients with vascular disease. In addition, new antithrombotic medications are likely to become available that will increase the precision and success of therapy.

REFERENCES

1. Schafer AI: The hypercoagulable states. *Ann Intern Med* 1985; 102:814–828.
2. Hart RG, Kanter MC: Hematologic disorders and ischemic stroke: A selective review. *Stroke* 1990; 21:1111–1121.
3. Coller BS, Owen J, Jasty J, et al: Deficiency of plasma protein S, protein C, or antithrombin III and arterial thrombosis. *Atherosclerosis* 1987; 7:456–462.
4. Clouse LH, Comp PC: The regulation of hemostasis: The protein C system. *N Engl J Med* 1986; 314:1298–1304.
5. Engesser L, Broekmans AW, Briet E, et al: Hereditary protein S deficiency: Clinical manifestations. *Ann Intern Med* 1987; 106:677–682.
6. Miletich J, Sherman L, Broze G: Absence of thrombosis in subjects with heterozygous protein C deficiency. *N Engl J Med* 1987; 317:991–996.
7. Mammen EF: Congenital coagulation disorders: Dysfibrinogenemia. *Semin Thromb Hemost* 1983; 9:4–9.
8. Aoki N, Moroi M, Sakata Y, et al: Abnormal plasminogen. A hereditary molecular abnormality found in a patient with recurrent thrombosis. *J Clin Invest* 1978; 61:1186–1195.
9. Soria J, Soria C, Bertrand O, et al: Plasminogen Paris I: Congenital abnormal plasminogen and its incidence in thrombosis. *Thromb Res* 1983; 32:229–238.
10. Stead NW, Bauer KA, Kinney TR, et al: Venous thrombosis in a family with defective release of vascular plasminogen activator and elevated plasma factor VIII/von Willebrand's factor. *Am J Med* 1983; 74:33–39.
11. O'Donnell TF, Carvalho ACA, Colman RW, et al: Platelet function abnormalities in a family with recurrent arterial thrombosis. *Surgery* 1978; 83:144–150.
12. McDaniel MD, Pearce WH, Yao JST, et al: Sequential changes in coagulation and platelet function following femorotibia bypass. *J Vasc Surg* 1984; 1:261–268.
13. Kluft C, Verheijen JH, Jie AFH, et al: The postoperative fibrinolytic shutdown: A rapidly reverting acute phase pattern for the fast-acting inhibitor of tissue-type plasminogen activator after trauma. *Scand J Clin Lab Invest* 1985; 45:605–610.
14. Davi G, Catalano I, Averna M, et al: Thromboxane biosynthesis and platelet function in type II diabetes mellitus. *N Engl J Med* 1990; 322:1769–1774.
15. Greenfield LJ: Lupus-like anticoagulants and thrombosis. *J Vasc Surg* 1988; 7::818–819.
16. Bacharach JM, Lie JT, Homburger HA: The prevalence of vascular occlusive disease associated with antiphospholipid syndromes. *Int Angiol* 1992; 11:51–56.
17. Asherson RA, Khamashta MA, Gil A, et al: Cerebrovascular disease and antiphospholipid antibodies in systemic lupus erythematosus, lupus-like disease, and the primary antiphospholipid syndrome. *Am J Med* 1989; 86:391–399.
18. Laster J, Cikrit D, Walker N, et al: The heparin-induced thrombocytopenia syndrome: An update. *Surgery* 1987; 102:763–770.
19. Kakkasseril JS, Cranley JJ, Panke T, et al: Heparin-induced thrombocytopenia: A prospective study of 142 patients. *J Vasc Surg* 1985; 2:382–384.
20. Laster J, Silver D: Heparin-coated catheters and heparin-induced thrombocytopenia. *J Vasc Surg* 1988; 7:667–672.
21. Mustard JF, Kinlough-Rathbone RL, Packham MA: The vessel wall in thrombosis, in Colman RW, Hirsh J, Marder VJ, et al (eds): *Hemostasis and Thrombosis—Basic Principles and Clinical Practice,* 2nd ed. Philadelphia, Lippincott, 1987, pp 1073–1088.
22. Fuster V, Badimon L, Badimon JJ, et al: The pathogenesis of coronary artery disease and the acute coronary syndromes. *N Engl J Med* 1992; 326:242–250.

23. Wu KK, Hoak JC: Increased platelet aggregates in patients with transient ischemic attacks. *Stroke* 1975; 6:521–524.
24. Taomoto K, Asada M, Kanzawa Y, et al: Usefulness of the measurement of plasma B-thromboglobulin (B-TG) in cerebrovascular disease. *Stroke* 1983; 14:518–524.
25. Trip MD, Cats VM, van Capelle FJL, et al: Platelet hyperreactivity and prognosis in survivors of myocardial infarction. *N Engl J Med* 1990; 322:1549–1554.
26. Donaldson MC, Matthews ET, Hadjimichael J, et al: Markers of thrombotic activity in arterial disease. *Arch Surg* 1987; 122:897–900.
27. McCollum CN, Kester RC, Rajah SM, et al: Arterial graft maturation: The duration of thrombotic activity in Dacron aortobifemoral grafts measured by platelet and fibrinogen kinetics. *Br J Surg* 1981; 68:61–64.
28. Marler JR, Price TR, Clark GL, et al: Morning increase in onset of ischemic stroke. *Stroke* 1989; 20:473–476.
29. Tofler GH, Brezinski D, Schafer AI, et al: Concurrent morning increase in platelet aggregability and the risk of myocardial infarction and sudden cardiac death. *N Engl J Med* 1987; 316:1514–1518.
30. Donaldson MC, Mannick JA, Whittemore AD: Causes of primary graft failure after in situ saphenous vein bypass grafting. *J Vasc Surg* 1992; 15:113–120.
31. Eldrup-Jorgensen J, Flanigan DP, Brace L, et al: Hypercoagulable states and lower limb ischemia in young adults. *J Vasc Surg* 1989; 9:334–341.
32. Hallet JW, Greenwood LH, Robison JG: Lower extremity arterial disease in young adults: A systematic approach to early diagnosis. *Ann Surg* 1985; 202:647–652.
33. Towne JB, Bandyk DF, Hussey CV, et al: Abnormal plasminogen: A genetically determined cause of hypercoagulability. *J Vasc Surg* 1984; 1:896–902.
34. Towne JB, Hussey CV, Bandyk DF: Abnormalities of the fibrinolytic system as a cause of upper extremity ischemia: A preliminary report. *J Vasc Surg* 1988; 7:661–666.
35. Shapiro ME, Rodvien R, Bauer KA, et al: Acute aortic thrombosis in antithrombin III deficiency. *JAMA* 1981; 245:1759–1761.
36. Karl R, Garlick I, Zarins C, et al: Surgical implications of antithrombin III deficiency. *Surgery* 1981; 89:429–433.
37. Towne JB, Bernhard VM, Hussey C, et al: Antithrombin deficiency—a cause of unexplained thrombosis in vascular surgery. *Surgery* 1981; 89:735–742.
38. Flinn WR, McDaniel MD, Yao JST, et al: Antithrombin III deficiency as a reflection of dynamic protein metabolism in patients undergoing vascular reconstruction. *J Vasc Surg* 1984; 1:888–895.
39. Baker WH, Potthoff WP, Biller J, et al: Carotid artery thrombosis associated with lupus anticoagulant. *Surgery* 1985; 98:612–615.
40. Shortell CK, Ouriel K, Green RM, et al: Vascular disease in the antiphospholipid syndrome: A comparison with the patient population with atherosclerosis. *J Vasc Surg* 1992; 15:158–166.
41. Ahn SS, Kalunian K, Rosove M, et al: Postoperative thrombotic complications in patients with the lupus anticoagulant: Increased risk after vascular procedures. *J Vasc Surg* 1988; 7:749–756.
42. Donaldson MC, Weinberg DS, Belkin M, et al: Screening for hypercoagulable states in vascular surgical practice: A preliminary study. *J Vasc Surg* 1990; 11:825–831.
43. Kappa JR, Fisher CA, Berkowitz HD, et al: Heparin-induced platelet activation in sixteen surgical patients: Diagnosis and management. *J Vasc Surg* 1987; 5:101–109.
44. Marciniak E, Gockerman JP: Heparin-induced decrease in circulating antithrombin III. *Lancet* 1977; 2:581–584.
45. Tuman KJ, McCarthy RJ, March RJ, et al: Effects of epidural anesthesia and

analgesia on coagulation and outcome after major vascular surgery. *Anesth Analg* 1991; 73:696–704.

46. Laster J, Elfrink R, Silver D: Re-exposure to heparin of patients with heparin-associated antibodies. *J Vasc Surg* 1989; 9:677–682.

47. Kappa JR, Cottrell ED, Berkowitz HD, et al: Carotid endarterectomy in patients with heparin-induced platelet activation: Comparative efficacy of aspirin and iloprost (ZK36374). *J Vasc Surg* 1987; 5:693–701.

48. Sobel M, Adelman B, Szentpetery S, et al: Surgical management of heparin-associated thrombocytopenia: Strategies in the treatment of venous and arterial thromboembolism. *J Vasc Surg* 1988; 8:395–401.

49. Makhoul RG, Greenberg CS, McCann RL: Heparin-associated thrombocytopenia and thrombosis: A serious clinical problem and potential solution. *J Vasc Surg* 1986; 4:522–528.

50. Cole CW, Bormanis J: Ancrod: A practical alternative to heparin. *J Vasc Surg* 1988; 8:59–63.

51. McCollum C, Alexander C, Kenchington G, et al: Antiplatelet drugs in femoropopliteal vein bypasses: A multicenter trial. *J Vasc Surg* 1991; 13:150–162.

52. Green RM, Roedersheimer LR, DeWeese JA: Effects of aspirin and dipyridamole on expanded polytetrafluoroethylene graft patency. *Surgery* 1982; 92:1016–1026.

53. Clyne CAC, Archer TJ, Atuhaire LK, et al: Random control trial of a short course of aspirin and dipyridamole (Persantine) for femorodistal grafts. *Br J Surg* 1987; 74:246–248.

54. Steering Committee of the Physicians' Health Study Research Group: Final report on the aspirin component of the ongoing physicians' health study. *N Engl J Med* 1989; 321:129–135.

55. Kretschmer G, Wenzl E, Piza F, et al: The influence of anticoagulant treatment on the probability of function in femoropopliteal vein bypass surgery: Analysis of a clinical series (1970 to 1985) and interim evaluation of a controlled clinical trial. *Surgery* 1987; 102:453–459.

56. Flinn WR, Rohrer MJ, Yao JST, et al: Improved long-term patency of infragenicular polytetrafluoroethylene grafts. *J Vasc Surg* 1988; 7:685–690.

Index

We've read
236,287
journal
articles

(so you don't have to).

The Year Books–
The best from 236,287 journal articles.

At Mosby, we subscribe to more than 950 medical and allied health journals from every corner of the globe. We read them all, tirelessly scanning for anything that relates to your field.

We send everything we find related to a given specialty to the distinguished editors of the **Year Book** in that area, and they pick out the best, the articles they feel every practitioner in that specialty should be aware of.

For the 1993 **Year Books** we surveyed a total of 236,287 articles and found hundreds of articles related to your field. Our expert editors reviewed these and chose the best, the developments you don't want to miss.

The best articles–condensed and organized.

Not only do you get the past year's most important articles in your field, you get them in a format that makes them easy to use.

Every article that the editors pick is condensed into a concise, outlined abstract, a summary of the article's most important points highlighted with bold paragraph headings. So you can quickly scan for exactly what you need.

Personal commentary from the experts.

If that was it, if all our editors did was identify the year's best articles, the **Year Book** would still be a great reference to have. (Can you think of an easier way to keep up with all the developments that are shaping your field?)

But following each article, the editors also write concise commentaries telling whether or not the study in question is a reliable one, whether a new technique is effective, or whether a particular trend you've heard about merits your immediate attention.

No other abstracting service offers this expert advice to help you decide how the year's advances will affect the way you practice.

No matter how many journals you subscribe to, the Year Book can help.

When you subscribe to a **Year Book**, we'll also send you an automatic notice of future volumes about two months before they publish. If you do not want the **Year Book**, this convenient advance notice makes it easy for you to let us know. And if you elect to receive the new **Year Book**, you need do nothing. We will send it upon publication.

No worry. No wasted motion. And, of course, every **Year Book** is yours to examine FREE of charge for thirty days.